FREE-HAND

DRAWING

"A MANUAL FOR TEACHERS AND STUDENTS"

By

ANSON K. CROSS

INSTRUCTOR IN THE MASSACHUSETTS NORMAL ART SCHOOL, AND IN THE SCHOOL OF DRAWING AND PAINTING, MUSEUM OF FINE ARTS, BOSTON; AUTHOR OF FREE-HAND DRAWING, LIGHT AND SHADE, AND FREE-HAND PERSPECTIVE, AND A SERIES OF TEXT AND DRAWING BOOKS FOR THE PUBLIC SCHOOLS.

ILLUSTRATED &

PUBLISHED BY

E-KİTAP PROJESİ & CHEAPEST BOOKS

www.cheapestboooks.com

Copyright, 2015 by e-Kitap Projesi Istanbul

ISBN:

978-625-6004-49-8

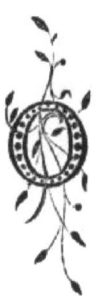

PREFACE.

THIS book is intended for public school teachers, and for all teachers and students of elementary drawing. Its object is the presentation of artistic methods of studying free-hand drawing.

In order that this book may be inexpensive, and may meet the needs of the large number of teachers whose instruction includes outline drawing only, light and shade, which is of interest to many teachers, is made the subject of another book.

An outline drawing is the most conventional of all pictorial methods of expression. It must often be incomplete, unsatis factory, and scientific, if not mechanical. There can be but one correct representation of a cube at any given distance level and angle, and an artistic outline drawing of a geometric model is often difficult if not impossible to produce.

There are, however, artistic and inartistic ways of making an outline drawing of a cube, and if such a drawing cannot be artistic, one drawing may be less mechanical than another, and may prepare the pupil to make artistic drawings of subjects which are easier to treat in this way than the exact drawing model. Many teachers think it impossible to give lessons in drawing without the use of mechanical methods, such as copying and dictating; but in some places public school instruction is artistic. It has been shown that it is easy to start correctly in the lower grades, and not impossible for the pupils of advanced grades to change from mechanical to artistic methods.

In order that this change may be made, it is not necessary that the teachers become artists, but that they give to the subject the time required to enable them to draw simple subjects correctly.

The methods presented have been tested in elementary and advanced schools, and, if followed, will give ability to draw correctly from nature in an artistic manner.

To secure satisfactory results it is necessary that those giving the most elementary instruction understand the requirements of more advanced work. For this reason the chapter on composition has been given, and no attempt has been made to arrange the book so that teachers may study simply the directions for their special grades.

ANSON K. CROSS.

INTRODUCTION.

A DRAWING is the expression of an idea : art must come from within, and not from without. This fact has led some to assert that the study of nature is not essential to the student, and that careful training in the study of the representation of the actual appearance is mechanical and harmful. Such persons forget that all art ideas and sentiments must be based upon natural objects, and that a person who cannot represent truly what he sees will be entirely unable to express the simplest ideal conceptions so that others may appreciate them. Study of nature is, then, of the first and greatest importance to the art student.

A drawing may be made in outline, in light and shade, or in color. The value of the drawing artistically, does not depend upon the medium used, but upon the individuality of the draughtsman making it. The simplest pencil sketch may have much more merit than an elaborate colored drawing made by one who is unable to represent truly the facts of nature, or who sees, instead of the beauty and poetry, the ugliness and the imperfections of the subject.

The value depends as little upon the way the medium is used as upon the medium chosen, providing of course that the technique is not unduly prominent or offensive. Those who assert that they have found the only medium fit to be used or the only satisfactory way of handling the medium, thus prove their ignorance of the subject which they attempt to teach.

The first question for the teacher is "Shall the pupil work in color, in light and shade, or in outline?" Color is, for the public schools at least, out of the question. Not only is it expensive, but impossible to teach. Until the students have been educated to see the actual colors of the spectrum, even the strongest artist, as teacher, would not be able to obtain satisfactory results, and for the public school teacher to attempt to teach form, light and shade, and color at first and at once is entirely beyond reason.

Choice of the drawing to be made lies between a light and shade and an outline drawing. For students outside the public schools, light and shade should be taken up as early as possible. After a few lessons in outline, a few in light and shade can be given, and the two lines of study may then be carried on together. In the public schools the study of light and shade at first or in the lower grades is unwise, and generally impossible to pursue with advantage to the pupils, for the reason that in the classroom it is almost impossible to get good light and shade upon objects placed so that they may be seen by the pupils. In the public schools the first instruction must then be in outline, and in the upper grades or the high schools, or whenever all the conditions are favorable, the study of light and shade may be begun.

CONTENTS.

FREE-HAND DRAWING.

CHAPTER I.

OUTLINE DRAWING.

An Outline Drawing may be made in many different ways. It may be drawn with the brush, charcoal, crayon, pen and ink, or pencil. The drawing is commonly made upon paper, although it may be made on other substances. The question for the teacher is "Which is the best medium for beginners to use?" The best medium is that which requires the least thought to handle and the least time to prepare and care for; it is that which allows the student to give all his attention to the comparison of his drawing with the object, and which admits most readily of changes. It is evident that the choice lies between charcoal and pencil, for the only value of the work is in the training and knowledge given by it. A charcoal drawing can be readily changed, but to provide this material for classes in the public schools would be very expensive, and the cause of very unclean schoolrooms. Crayon and colored chalk have no advantage over pencil: on the contrary they are more expensive, and a drawing made with them cannot be changed except with great difficulty. The pencil is not only cheaper and neater, but it requires less time to sharpen, and when rightly used the correct lines can be obtained without any erasing; so that this simple means is really the best for educational purposes.

When the crayon, red chalk, pen and ink, or the brush is used in the lower grades, the probabilities are that the aim of the instruction given is for something to exhibit, instead of for the best education.

The pencil will make a drawing with an amount of finish and effect, ranging from an outline of the simplest nature to a rendering of all the values of a complicated subject; and when it is understood that the only worth of the drawing lies in the truthfulness with which it represents nature, we shall find childish attempts to handle difficult mediums less frequent than at present.

It is often said that there are no outlines in nature. In a way this is true, but it cannot be understood to mean that form is unnecessary or that it may be slighted. The student cannot learn to paint or to make pictures in any medium, without drawing the forms of the objects. The defining of the lights and shades and the various bits of color which are seen in nature is necessary to give solidity and character to a picture, and it is useless to think that anything can be accomplished with color or light and shade if approximate representations of form cannot be made.

Every object has definite form and size, and though it may not be outlined, it has boundaries. Although the representation of objects in outline is at best a conventional and imperfect means of expression, so far often as even form is concerned, the student can be taught to observe effects, and may often succeed in conveying a fair impression of the character of the object, and of varieties of surface and texture. He will find that the study of appearances, and their representation as fully as possible, even in so simple a way as outline drawing, will in a great measure prepare the way for work in light and shade and color. The whole question is simply one of seeing, and the student should not trouble himself over technique, as his only aim should be a true representation of nature, and it is of no consequence that such drawings by different people may be produced in different ways.

The most important points in free-hand drawing are freedom, directness, and accuracy. It is difficult to give directions which will produce these results, as individuality will prevent all from working in a uniform way. It is necessary, however, to give general directions for the work, and especially to advise the pupil not to follow the directions given in many books, written by those who are not artists or draughtsmen.

Chapter I. presents the general information required by art students and all teachers, even those of the most elementary work. Special directions are given in following chapters in order that the most important facts may be presented first.

GENERAL DIRECTIONS.

First, the surface on which the drawing is made must be held so that it is at right angles to the direction in which it is seen. If the book or paper is placed upon the desk, and the pupil looks down obliquely at it, the drawing upon it must be foreshortened so that it is impossible for the student to see what he is doing.

If the drawing is upon a block or upon paper placed upon a board, it may be held at the proper angle by the left hand. If the drawing is made in a drawing book, the book must be fastened to a stiff piece of cardboard or a thin drawing board, so that it may be properly held.

Second, the paper or book should be held as far as possible from the eyes. The student should sit back in the chair, and holding the pencil very lightly, should suggest or indicate the position of the drawing upon the paper by light lines, drawn quickly with a movement of the entire arm from the shoulder. Before beginning to draw, the student should practise this free arm movement by drawing horizontal, vertical, and oblique lines. These lines should be drawn and redrawn, the arm passing rapidly along the paper, and the pencil point tracing line after line as near the first one as possible.

After the straight line movement, circular and elliptical movements should be practised in the same way. These exercises should be repeated by the students whenever they have a moment not occupied, until they can sweep in an approximate ellipse, or circle, or draw a straight line with one light, quick stroke of the arm.

The pencil should be long, of medium grade, and should be held by the thumb and first two fingers, with its unsharpened end directed toward the palm of the hand. It should be held in this way for all the first work upon any drawing, but in finishing or accenting a drawing whose lines have been thus sketched, more pressure will be required, and the pencil may be held nearer the point.

If the drawing is made upon a sheet of paper, it should be secured to the board by tacks, so that its edges are parallel to those of the board; if the edges are not quite straight, a horizontal line may be drawn near the lower edge, so that directions may be referred to this line.

If the drawing is made in a book, the directions, vertical and horizontal, will be obtained by comparison with the edges of the book.

DRAWING FROM SINGLE OBJECTS.

We will suppose that the subject of our lesson is the box, Fig. 1.

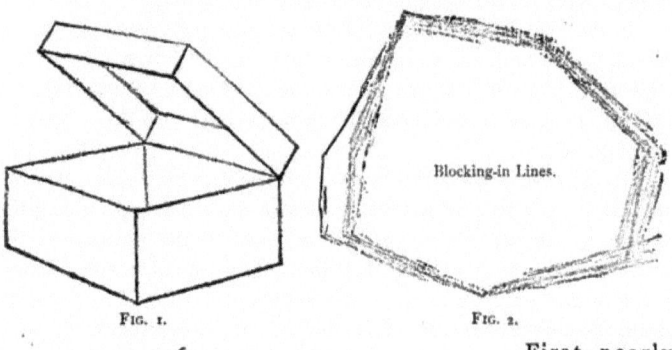

Blocking-in Lines.

Fig. 1.   Fig. 2.

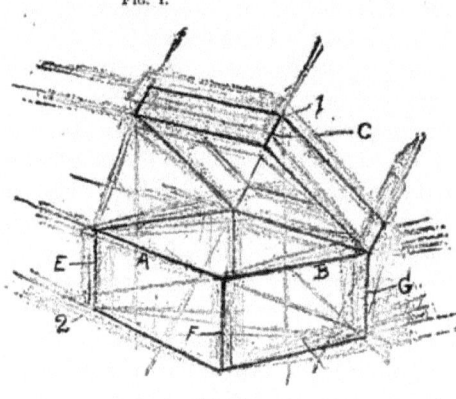

Fig. 3.

First, nearly close the eyes and try to see the box not as a solid, but as a silhouette. The pupils will understand what is desired if an object is held in front of a window, for they will then see the object as a mass of dark, whose outlines are very distinct, while the lines within the contour are almost, if not quite, invisible. Practice will enable one to look at all objects so as to think simply of the directions of their outer lines.

To realize the directions which the important lines appear to have, the pencil point may be moved back and forth in the air so that it appears to cover the edges. In other words, the lines may be drawn in the air. While doing this care should be taken to keep the pencil point where it would be if it were held upon a pane of glass placed in front of the pupil, and at right angles to the direction in which the object is seen, and not to move the pencil away from the eyes, that is, in the actual direction of the edges. This test is the most valuable of all, because it is the simplest and easiest to apply. It is really the same as the use of the thread, explained on page 47, and nearly all other means of testing will at last be discarded in favor of this first and simplest.

After careful study of the mass, its outline may be lightly sketched, no measurements of proportion having been made. The aim is to train the eye to see correctly. In order to do this, the student must depend upon his eye, and put down its first impression, rather than the results of mechanical tests of proportions. He must first draw, and then test by measuring.

The suggesting of the mass of the drawing by light, quick lines, serves to place the drawing to the best advantage on the paper, and to introduce the draughtsman to the problem before him and to the means by which it is to be worked out. These lines are called blocking-in lines, and from such illustrations as Fig. 4, which is suggested by the cuts of a book on drawing, pupils are often led to think that a great deal of time must

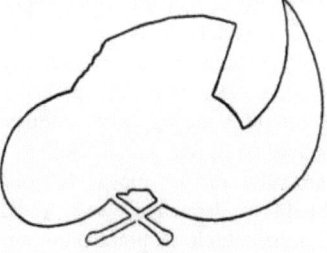

Fig. 4. Unsatisfactory Blocking-in Lines.

be spent on the lines, that they must be nicely drawn, and that every little indentation or change of form in the outline of the mass must be carefully given. Such ideas are productive of much harm. These lines should be put in lightly and freely, and should do no more than give the proportions of the drawing and its position upon the paper.

When the outline of the mass has been suggested, the inner lines may be indicated, and the result carefully studied to see that it agrees with the appearance. When no more can be done by eye alone, the drawing may be tested by measuring the proportions as explained in Chapter V.   If the sketch does not agree with these tests, it must be changed.   All changes should be made, not by erasing, but by drawing new lines, and the drawing should be carried on in this way, until the correct lines are obtained.

The first lines must be very light.   As changes are made, the strength may be increased to distinguish them, until the correct line is secured.   The drawing having been changed to agree with

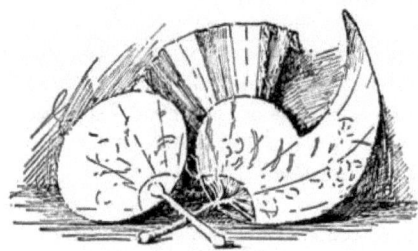

FIG. 5.   The explanation of Fig. 4.

the measurements of the whole height and width, and tested by moving the pencil point to cover the edges, it will be well to test it by means of vertical and horizontal lines taken through the different angles of the box.   Thus, drop the pencil point vertically from point 1, and see where it cuts the lower edge; carry the point horizontally from point 2, and note its intersection with the front edge.   The pencil may now be made to continue the apparent directions of the edges A, B, C, etc., until the points where the continued lines appear to intersect the opposite outlines are noted.   Such tests may also be applied by the pencil used as a straight edge, held horizontally, vertically, and to appear to coincide with the lines.   These tests should be depended upon, and if carefully made, will produce a drawing which is practically correct.   The first measurements of height and width should be very carefully taken.   Distances which are nearly equal, as EF and FG, may also be compared; but as a rule, few measurements of proportion should be made, as short distances, or short with long distances, cannot be compared with sufficient accuracy to be of any value.

Instead of the pencil the thread may be used for testing, as explained on page 47.   The thread appears a fine line, whose intersections with the edges may be easily placed, so that until the eye can be depended upon, the thread is preferable to the pencil.

It is most important that all changes be made not by erasing, but by drawing new lines. Erasing and keeping but one line from first to last will generally produce a hard and inaccurate drawing; and although it may finally be made to agree with all the tests, it will be lacking in spirit. It is difficult at first for most students to draw lightly enough to secure the correct lines without too great heaviness, but it is better, rather than to erase, to throw the drawing away and start anew, until the result can be secured without having lines so black that they cannot easily be erased.

The reason for working in this way is that we wish the student to depend, as far as possible, on his eyes. If he erases and has only one line from the start, unnecessary time is given to the drawing, and he will hesitate to change his lines. If light lines are drawn and not erased, but others drawn as soon as there is doubt about the first being rightly placed, the student is much more free to change as each suggestion occurs, and toward the last he has his choice of the various lines already drawn and can experiment freely.

This is by far the quickest and most accurate way, and prepares for rapid and truthful sketching. It is difficult at first for the student who has been taught the mechanical way of drawing one line at a time, but he will not have to draw very long in this way before he will be able to produce truthful sketches without drawing many unnecessary lines.

The student has simply to study the sketches and drawings made by the old masters, and also those by the artists and illustrators of the present day, to perceive that this is the way in which artists draw, and to see that with them, the first light touches generally remain and become part of the finished drawing.

Some artists are able to draw at first touch so as to give exact proportions to everything, but this power is due to long study resulting in thorough knowledge and ability to see correctly. This knowledge is easiest and best attained by the process of considering the subject as a whole, by suggesting all the parts at once, and then of bringing them into their proper relations as described.

In making an outline drawing pupils must erase all the first lines; and if they are not able to obtain the correct lines without getting the paper so black that it cannot be readily cleaned, there is no reason why a hard pencil should not be used for the sketching. This outline work is simply educational, and certainly at first is not artistic. If a hard pencil is used very lightly, its marks may be removed without smooching, and the lines may be shifted a great many times without any injury to the paper. When the pupils draw more correctly, they will be able to draw the first suggestive lines with the soft pencil, which should be used in accenting the drawings.

When the correct outline has been found, it is necessary for the pupils to erase all unnecessary lines. The easiest way to do this and still retain the correct lines is to make them stronger than the others so that they will show faintly when the eraser has been passed over the paper, removing all but an indication of the desired result.

The drawing may then be accented. A soft pencil should be used, held more firmly and nearer the point. The lines should be drawn of their proper strength at one touch, and no attempt should be made to get them absolutely uniform. Much time is often wasted in such attempts, and the tendency is for too much importance to be put upon the character of the line, and too little upon the form expressed by the line. In the first work it is not necessary to think of the line, as the objects are geometric, and there is little chance for artistic effects. If the lines are put in at one touch, they will be much more satisfactory artistically than if the students are allowed to labor over them for any effect whatever.

Especially to be avoided is the smooth, even line which has the effect of having been drawn with the ruler. These lines are so inartistic that we often find labored attempts to avoid the mechanical effects due to their use. The "broad gray line," which ought from its name to be much better than the fine even line, is often more unsatisfactory, for certain valuable training results from the making of fine regular lines. No knowledge of drawing is necessary to make the "broad gray line"; yet some seem to think this quality of line the only attribute of a good drawing, and so important that it must be obtained even at the expense of drawing two lines and carefully filling in the space between them.

The width and character of the lines are unimportant as long as they are freely drawn and express the appearance of the object.

When pupils are able to draw correctly, it will be necessary only to ask them to work as simply and directly as possible, and to make drawings which are strong and effective at a distance. To do this, they must use a soft pencil when accenting, and accent at one touch.

If the lines are put in at one touch, they will be slightly irregular and varied, and will give a satisfactory result; for in a free-hand drawing representing even the geometric solids that have keen, sharp edges, lines which are ruled, or which are drawn free-hand to look like ruled lines, are very unsatisfactory: they produce a mechanical drawing. An artistic drawing must have variety, and must even represent sharp straight lines by lines which are not perfectly smooth and regular. This is according to the way we see these lines in Nature, for the influence of the atmosphere, which is always vibrating, causes the lines to appear not quite straight. Vibration is seen in the glittering lines of the railway track, which in summer through the hot rays of the noon-day sun seem to quiver and dance about. This and similar effects will often be seen by the student of Nature.

The pupil is frequently told to finish his drawing in lines which are strong for the parts near the eye, and lines which are light for the parts farther away. Such accenting is a mechanical application of a principle which is true and necessary in good work, but when applied without judgment to any subject, it produces the most hard and mechanical results, and students should never be allowed to accent by this or any other rule. To make an outline drawing which is artistic in its effect is a very difficult problem. It cannot be solved by the young pupil, and for the first work it is better to use lines of uniform strength and to say nothing about accenting, than it is to give a rule, or to attempt what is beyond the students' power to see and feel.

When the pupils are able to represent simple geometric forms correctly and readily, these may be arranged in groups.

DRAWING FROM GROUPS.

The student who has not had the best instruction will probably attempt to draw the objects one at a time, taking first the prism *A*, Fig. 6, next the vase *B*, then the cylinder *C*, and last the frame *D*.

The objection to this way of proceeding is that as the objects are drawn one at a time, until the last is completed, the proportion of the whole group — that is, its greatest height in comparison with its greatest width — cannot be seen. Indeed, this is often not even considered, the student taking it for granted that, since he measured and tested each object as it was drawn, the single objects are

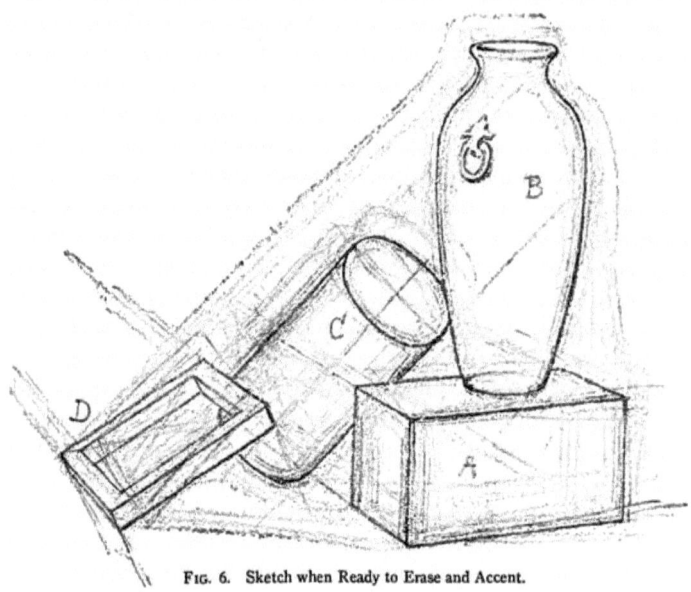

FIG. 6.   Sketch when Ready to Erase and Accent.

correct, and therefore the group. But each object is likely to be a little out of proportion; indeed, we may say is sure to be so. This being the case, the errors are multiplied; and if the whole height and width are compared, the proportion is found to be far from correct.

The whole should be presented before its parts, and drawing the different objects of the group one at a time, until finally the patch-work is complete, is an uneducational way of proceeding. Practically it is also most unsatisfactory, as with each object the difficulties increase, and at last it becomes impossible to place the drawings where they belong. The only logical way is to draw the group all at once, first considering it as a mass and blocking in its proportions by lines passing from the principal points, as in Fig. 7. When these lines have been drawn and considered, they may be tested by measuring the whole height and width, and the directions tested by use of the thread or pencil; but these lines must not follow at all closely the short lines upon the contour of the group. Their only legitimate purpose is to place the drawing properly upon the paper, and to give the extreme points of the drawing.

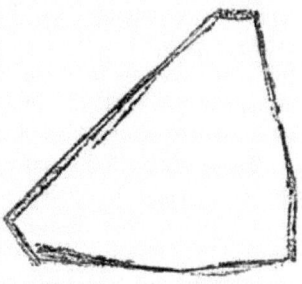

FIG. 7. Blocking-in Lines.

A good plan is, as soon as the proportions have been thus determined, to draw horizontal and vertical lines to indicate the upper, lower, right and left points of the drawing, and to be careful that the drawing is kept within these lines. The proportions of the whole group being thus determined as nearly as measurements can determine, the objects may now be sketched by eye, the most important lines being drawn first. These are the lines whose positions and directions are most easily seen. They are the longest lines, lines of one object which are nearly continuations of those of some other object, and lines which are brought out distinctly by shadow. It is evident that in this way the drawings of the different objects are proceeding at the same time, and, the shorter and less prominent lines being drawn last, the group may be said to be drawn all at once, or as if it were a single object having many parts.

While drawing, the student must think of the tests applied by the thread, of horizontal and vertical lines, and of continued lines; and drawing in the air, by moving the pencil point to hide the edges to be represented, will also help greatly. The object should be studied in this way and changed as often as found incorrect, until the eye can do no more. It is now time to apply systematically the tests explained by the drawings of the box, Fig. 1.

The first test is to compare the height and width of each object of the group, and also to compare these dimensions with those of the whole group. This test is the most important and should be very carefully taken. Slight inaccuracy can hardly be avoided, but the longest measurements can be compared more accurately than any others, especially in the case of those which are nearly equal, and the best that can be done is to make the drawing agree with these measurements. By this time the student should be able to measure as accurately as drawings of this nature require.

These tests will generally change the drawing throughout. The changes should be made, not by erasing, but by adding lines, until without other measurements the eye can see no more to be done. The thread may then be used, first for the tests of horizontal and vertical lines, second for the continuing of all the edges, and third for covering points in the group opposite one another, that the intersections of these lines with the edges may be noted. The thread used thus will discover every discrepancy except the slight deviations which only the accurate eye can detect. The training which is given by making drawings entirely by eye and then applying tests will soon produce power to draw correctly without the use of tests.

When the correct lines have been found, the others are to be erased, as explained on page 8, and the drawing is to be accented. But now the student will do well to think of effect, and to see if more interest and expression cannot be given to the drawing than is given by uniform lines. The student has perhaps been taught that the nearest objects are seen most strongly, and that the strength diminishes with the distance. This of course is true in a general way. It is the effect of aerial perspective, or the changing of color by intervening atmosphere. Thus, of a row of light objects the nearest will appear the lightest and brightest, and of a number of dark objects the nearest will appear the darkest. The light object in the distance appears darker,[1] and the dark one lighter, and in a sketch representing considerable distance this principle will be of assistance ; but it must be stated so as not to convey the idea that there can be nothing in the distance as strong or stronger than the unimportant features of the foreground, for we do not see objects

---

[1] Very light objects may change but little.

more or less distinctly according to their distance,— in fact, distance has practically nothing to do with it. *We distinguish objects as masses of color, lighter or darker than the colors against which they are seen.* This being so, it is evident that a light object in the background, as a white house seen against dark foliage, must be much more prominent than a near object, seen against another of the same color.

In general, when there is little or no contrast of color, objects are difficult to see without regard to their distance. Place a square of white cardboard in front of a larger square of the same, the latter coming in front of the blackboard. The smaller can be seen very faintly. In comparison with the distinctness with which the larger is seen against the blackboard, the smaller is practically invisible. This experiment proves that we distinguish objects through contrasts of color, and we have to consider what can be done in mere outline to render the effect of Nature. Can no more be done than to represent the form by lines of uniform strength?

The opinion seems to be general that more can be done. We find that instruction is often given to represent the nearer edges by strong lines, the farther ones by light lines; in fact, to proportion the strength of the line to the distance of the part it represents. Apply this rule to the representation of the two pieces of cardboard, and the nearer is accented by heavy lines, the farther by light lines. This is a direct contradiction of what we see, for the outline of the nearer is barely visible, while the farther is distinct against the blackboard.

In color we certainly should not think of representing the nearer as darker than the farther, or in any other way than as it appears, and the same is true of light and shade. Why should we not do the same *when possible*, with outline? No reason to the contrary can be given, for the difference in clearness with which the various lines are seen is the result, not of distance, but of contrasts of color, and light and shade. Of course we shall expect to find the strongest lines among the nearest ones, but farther than this we cannot go, and if we adopt any conventional accenting, we are working by rule and not by observation, and the result will be the production of hard, mechanical drawings.

Character appears in outlines. An object, as a cast, having a smooth, hard surface, shows these qualities in its outlines, which will be represented by relatively smooth lines. A cube with smooth faces has sharp, straight edges, which will be represented by straight lines. A box made of rough boards has broken edges, whose character may be given by drawing the irregular outline in which one surface breaks into the other. A drawing from the figure can express the variations in the appearance of the outline, parts of which are sharp, other parts blurred by light or a growth of hair.

Light affects the appearance of the outlines strongly, in some places making them distinct, in other places indistinct. An even line for everything disregards all these variations of effect; so also does any conventional variation of strength. If the student is allowed to disregard effects in outline work, he will have great difficulty in seeing them in later work. There is no more labor involved in representing effects than in disregarding them, for one line is as easy to make as another, *observation only being required. The student who can see, can in time* represent what he sees, and as long as any differences can be found between his drawing and Nature, he can learn to correct the errors.

The conventional accenting taught in many public schools produces the most mechanical, hard, and unnatural sketches when the student works from Nature, indoors or out. Undirected he would never produce such childish and ridiculous effects, but after instruction in drawing, which has specified that lines must be represented with a degree of strength corresponding to their distance, he naturally does not think of observing and drawing what he sees, but simply mechanically grades the strength of line as he has been taught. He makes the heaviest lines of the drawing where there should be the faintest indications of lines, and often where no lines at all would be better than faint ones.

It is almost impossible to get a pupil from most public schools to make sketches in which the unimportant detail, which is no part of the effect, is not brought out with heavy black lines. This is not surprising, for he sees this detail and it is near him, therefore, according to his instruction, it must be strongly accented.

In outline, as in other mediums, we should do the best we can to express what is before us. The effect of the subject should be considered as well as its form. There is no reason why the student should not be taught to observe the effect, and if once started rightly he will advance rapidly and will make drawings which, since they are representations of Nature, will have variety of effect, will be true and artistic. *No rule for accenting can be given* other than to study and represent what is seen, as far as possible, as it appears.

In outline, without any light and shade, it is impossible always to accent the lines just as they appear. For instance, some edges of

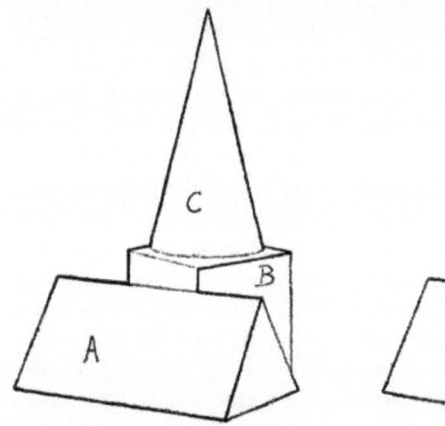 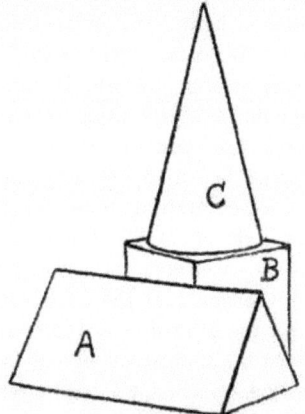

FIG. 8. Incorrectly Accented.   FIG. 9. Correctly Accented.

the object may be so lost in the shadow as to be wholly invisible, but without them the drawing might be incomplete and unsatisfactory. *A correct impression of the facts must be conveyed*, and no important line of a visible surface can be omitted even if not seen. Thus, in a brick or other building, when the light comes from directly behind the spectator, and the walls of the building are foreshortened equally, the front edge of the building will be invisible, unless it is brought out by different material or color. In an outline sketch of the building it would be necessary to represent this invisible edge, and it might be necessary to represent it by a very strong line, since the edge is the nearest line of the building. Thus the judgment and good sense of the draughtsman must decide what will give the best impression of the facts that the medium is capable of rendering.

In drawings of the geometric solids, where there are few lines, it will often be impossible to accent the lines as they appear; for some of the most important ones may be invisible, or seen so faintly that to represent them as they appear would make the drawing give a false impression. Frequently when the objects are strongly lighted and arranged as in Fig. 8, their outlines on the light side of the group intersect one another, so that the outline of the mass is composed of parts of those of several objects. This outline is very prominent, while the edges inside the outline are almost lost in the mass of light. It is evident that in this case we cannot accent as we see. We must accent as we feel the group, and when accenting the lines as they are seen is unsatisfactory, we must use our judgment and make the accenting express the facts. In Fig. 8, for instance, we must show that the prism A is in front of the cube B, and that the cone C is a solid and comes in front of the back faces of the cube.

When drawing from furniture or from any subject having many lines, the effect will often be satisfactory when the lines are accented as they are seen. Here there are so many lines and so many changes in direction that the parts which are not seen may not be missed, and the student can represent more nearly what he sees. But it must be understood that it is wholly a matter of feeling for which no rule can be given, and often, in such a case as that illustrated in Fig. 10, if the lines are accented as they appear, a very false idea of the facts will be conveyed, and instead of outlining the forms of the different parts going to make up the object, the outlines of the different spaces or bits of background seen between the various parts of the object will be given.

In drawing, these spaces should be considered, and their proportions will help to prove the work; but in accenting they are unimportant. It is important to give the form and position of the different pieces forming the object, and this must be done by the accenting in heavy lines of the important features. In such accenting, the student must remember that the heaviest accent or line will strike the eye first, and should thus be given to the nearest and most important parts, as in Fig. 11.

At first most students will have difficulty in seeing any difference in the way in which the various edges appear. This is due to the fact that but a single point can be seen clearly at any one time. The eye glances rapidly over the whole of an object, observing all its parts. We are unconscious of this motion. All parts of the object are seen distinctly, and the variety of effect is not realized. All the parts will continue to give the impression of equal strength until the ability to see the whole of an object at once has been acquired. The student must practise until he can thus see before he thinks of success in any medium, for all demand equally a study of the comparative strength of detail.

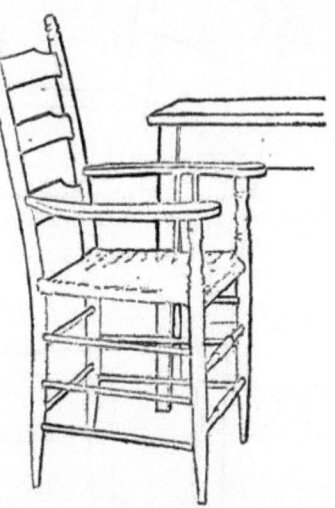

FIG. 10. Incorrectly Accented.

It is almost impossible for students to realize effects and masses. The best assistance in this direction is given by the use of an ordinary magnifying glass of about 12" or 15" focus. If the pupil hold this as far from him as he can and still see in it the blurred forms of the group he is studying, he will see, if his eyes are focussed on the glass and not on the group, the masses of light and dark and color which form the effect, and which he must represent if his drawing is to be true. This glass is called a blur-glass, because it blurs away the detail which the pupil exaggerates so much as to spoil his drawing. If this glass is used in light and shade and in color work, it will prove the best teacher the pupil can have. In outline work, it will enable pupils to see the difference in the effect of the different lines. After using this glass for a short time, the pupils will learn to see the whole of the group at once by looking at it with the eyes out of focus, and they will not require the blur-glass to realize the effects they ought to represent.

It is not possible to see simply, to realize effects and masses, without the blurred vision, which gives an impression of the whole subject

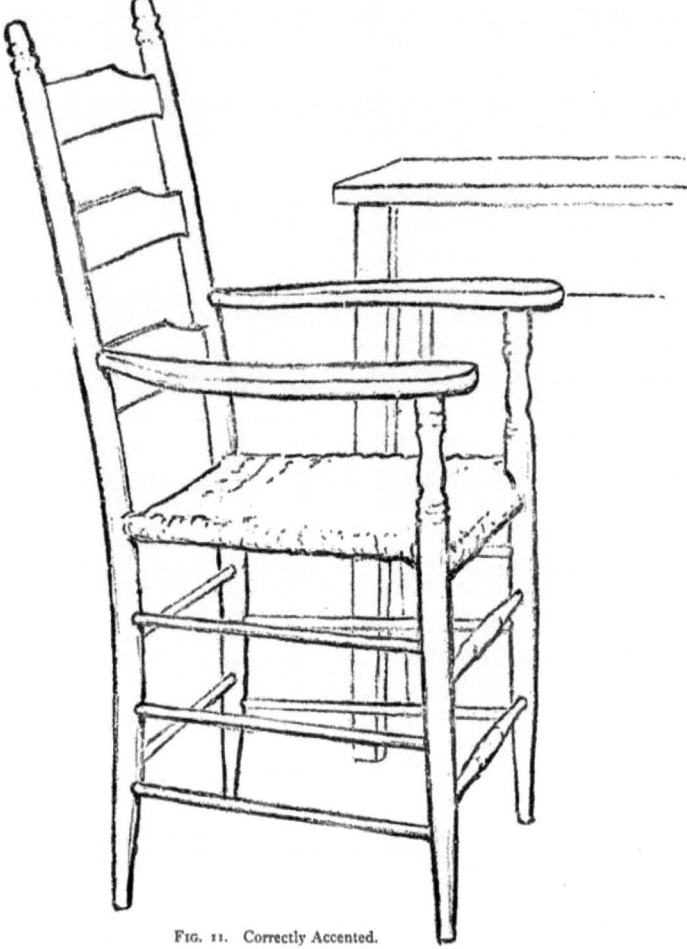

Fig. 11.   Correctly Accented.

at once.   No injury to the eyes results from proper blurring of vision
by a blur-glass, but if pupils try to look through it instead of at it,
they injure the sight and fail to see the masses.

Although no rule for accenting can be given, the effect is found to conform to the principle that *any detail which comes in either the mass of the light or that of the shadow is unimportant.* Thus an edge defining a light surface against another surface also light is not prominent, and an edge separating a surface in the shadow from another shade surface is seen faintly. The important features are those which come between the light and the shadow. But from what has been said it will be realized that an outline drawing is most conventional, and that the representation of what is really seen of outline will often be most unsatisfactory. The contour of an object is absolute, and an outline will give what the eye sees; but to express in outline artistically the pupil must learn to feel, and this cannot be expected at first. All that one can say to the student is observe the object, and do what is seen when this does not contradict the facts.

The following suggestions may aid pupils to accent satisfactorily:

1. The difference in distance of the different objects or the different parts of the same object, should be expressed by varied accenting, in which the strong lines represent important lines of the subject.

2. The strongest accents should represent the nearest important lines of the subject.

3. The lines of the background or any unimportant detail should be represented by light lines.

4. The forms of the different objects and their different parts, instead of those of the background seen behind the objects or between its different parts, must be brought out by the accenting.

The student will often, of his own accord, break away from outline pure and simple, and introduce light and shade features. This should be allowed and recommended in the public schools as soon as the pupils are able to make fairly correct outline drawings, and to see the shadows which may serve as accents. In the drawing of the geometric objects, unless the entire light and shade effects are given, it will not be easy to improve the drawing in this way; but in the study of common objects, or flowers and foliage, and of furniture, there will be many small cast shadows which can be seen and represented by the pupils. Even in an outline drawing these cast shadows can be expressed by a thickening of the line, and the earlier the students represent all important features that they can see, the easier it will be for them to make artistic drawings.   The drawings of the shoe and stool illustrate work of this nature, which is principally outline, and in which the cast shadows are given or suggested, and serve as accents.

The next step after the addition of small cast shadows is the rendering of the masses of light and dark : this introduces "Light and Shade," the subject of another book.

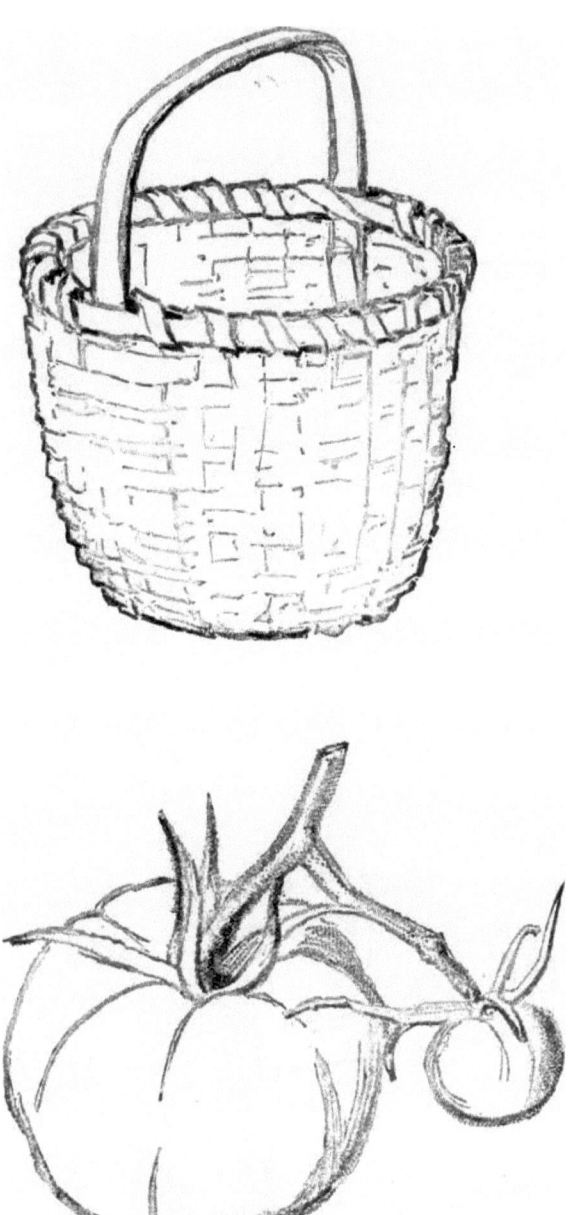

From the National Drawing Books.

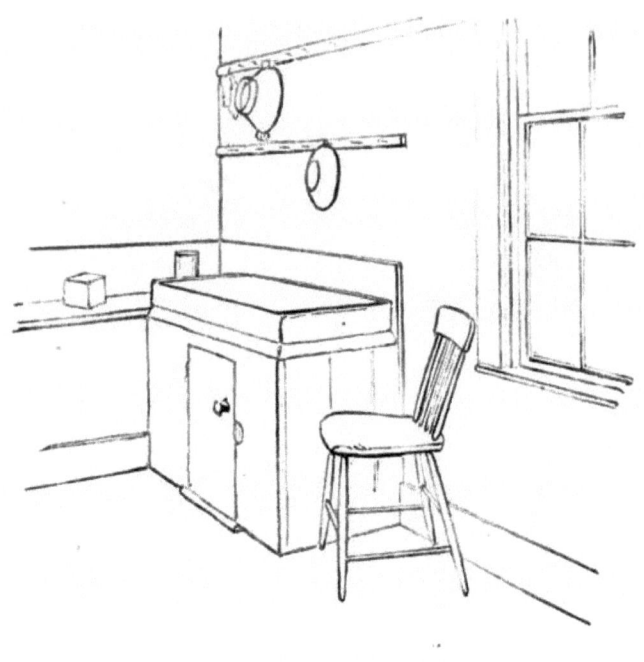

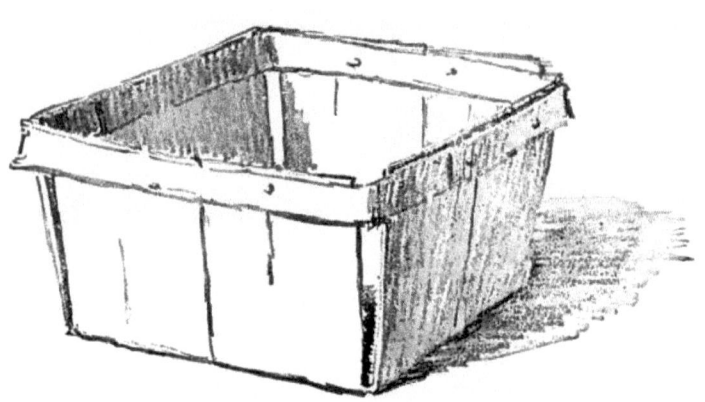

From the National Drawing Books.

CHAPTER II.

OBJECTS FOR STUDY.

WE hear a great deal now about the cultivation of the sense of beauty by the choice of drawing models. Many go so far as to say that nothing but the most beautiful forms should be given from the start, and, asserting that the cube, cylinder, and other type forms are not beautiful, they say that they should not be used, but that beautiful variations of these type forms should be provided. More definite information than this is rarely given. We are not told what natural objects are beautiful, and cheap enough to be provided, or how these objects of beauty are to be obtained, if they are not provided by the city. Such advice as to the use of beautiful models must be very pleasant and valuable to the drawing teacher, who so often fails to secure the money necessary to provide the cheap wooden models costing a few cents each ; and we do not wonder that special and regular teachers often regard this subject as one having no standards and no authorities.

Much of all this commotion about beautiful objects of study is raised by those who, suffering from criticism, have in the desire to escape it plunged headlong from one set of mechanical rules for a series of lessons for the public schools, to another set less arbitrary in certain directions, but still mechanical, and if possible, more harmful than before, because attempting more.

The average teacher can readily learn to discover at a glance whether or not the drawing of a cube represents the object as it might appear. She can do this even without seeing the model from the pupil's position; and the student can compare his drawing with the object and discover its errors more easily than he can in the drawing of a cast, a leaf, a figure, or any other object of beauty, in which the beauty depends upon lines which are subtle and which require a trained eye to see at all truly.

It is absurd to think that a pupil will profit by taking for his first lessons the most difficult problems. He may be satisfied, and generally is better satisfied, to make drawings which are childish attempts at work beyond his perception, than to begin the severe study of the elements of his art; but if he is serious and begins by attempting to produce pictures, he will always come at last to the study of the alphabet, namely, form and values. I have yet to know an artist of reputation who does not say that corrections of errors in drawing and in light and shade, or color effects, are the most important work of the teacher: in fact, are the greater part of what the teacher can do for the pupil.

Any drawing which does not help the student to make a better one has not properly educated him. To be helpful, the drawing must be criticised, and any teacher who gives her students work which she cannot criticise, must retard their progress. If public school teachers were generally able to criticise figure drawing and drawings from the most refined and beautiful forms, supposing that these forms could be provided and were best for the pupils to study, they would be unable to give their classes instruction in drawing for lack of time. When forty pupils are to be instructed in fifteen or twenty minutes, each can have but an instant of individual attention; and with objects of the nature of those recommended, the most skilful artist would not be able to criticise the work of one quarter of the class.

But these objects are not only impossible to obtain and difficult to work from, but they are really not as desirable, educationally, as the now despised cube, cylinder, etc. The best education is due to individual effort: particularly in drawing is this true. The student can criticise the errors in the drawing of the cube, and thus can help himself. The teacher can carry the criticism farther, and at a glance can say whether the drawing is correct; for there is but one possible appearance of a cube at a given distance, level, and angle. There is but one cube — that is, but one type form. Of potatoes and other similar forms there is no type, every object is individual, and therefore every consideration proves the cube and other geometric objects the best material for study. All of any experience know that those who can draw these objects and their variations easily and accurately, can draw almost anything. The students who begin by studying objects whose drawings they cannot criticise, and which, as has been shown, cannot be criticised for them, are not likely to progress far or well; and though study from natural or artistic variations of the solids is interesting and valuable, this should not come first nor be given exclusively until the more severe forms can be drawn easily and correctly. Not only for young pupils, but for all beginning the study of drawing, are the geometric forms the best objects of instruction. Properly studied, more ability in drawing will be gained from them in a given time than from any other material. The student who has drawn from life, even for many years, will find the drawing of geometric forms not only interesting, but valuable, because they will often prove to him that they are difficult to draw and that he cannot draw them well or easily. The student who can draw one thing well ought to be able to draw another; but many draw from memory as much or even more than from the object, and those who have not studied these forms are without the training which is most valuable for all work in which perspective is involved.

Groups including the double cross and the various frames are very difficult to draw, for they present many problems in foreshortening and the slightest error in drawing is very noticeable. For these reasons, all public school instruction should be based upon the geometric type forms. It may be said that to make the children interested in the subject of drawing, interesting subjects must be given them, and that in the continued drawing of the severe type forms they will lose their interest. Under the usual conditions, in which it is necessary for pupils to depend wholly upon the teachers for the correction of their work, students may not be interested in geometric subjects; but if they are enabled to correct their own drawings, they will find these subjects interesting, for they will see the value derived from each lesson.

In the first work it is much better to have the pupils draw from models placed upon their own desks than from objects farther away, for the reason that there is more perspective effect and the drawings are easier to criticise. When small models are placed at the back of each desk, the pictorial effect is not pleasant, as there is too violent perspective; but this effect may be avoided by placing the models upon the model support, books, or some other object which will raise them a few inches from the desk. This first work, however, cannot be pictorially pleasing or artistic. It must be educational, and considered in this light the position of the models on the desk is the best that can be found for the first work, since they are near the pupil, and he can test his drawings very exactly, much more easily and better than he could were the models at a greater distance. Another advantage is that the pupils are independent, and may advance as rapidly as they are able. Those who finish a drawing, instead of waiting for those who have not finished, can rearrange the model and draw again. The simple tablets and solids are thus adapted to give the most severe and valuable training to the pupils. After study from them for a short time, they will be able to see correctly enough to make good drawings from objects of common use and interest.

The best models for the first work in the public schools consist of cardboard tablets which may be connected by means of metal clips, or by rods fitting sockets secured to the tablets. The tablets are sold in sets, including the common geometric forms, and by combining them the solid type forms may be represented in whole or in part. The chief value of these models over the wooden models is due to the fact that by their use, the edges of the solids which are invisible may be made visible, for the tablets may be combined to present the appearance of the interior, as well as that of the exterior of the solid forms. By connecting the bases of the prism forms by a rod, these forms are presented to the pupils in the simplest way. When thus arranged all, or nearly all, of the angles of two or more type forms, arranged in a group, may be seen at the same time. These models are thus much easier to draw correctly than the solid objects.

The metal clips hold the tablets at right angles to each other, but they may be bent to give any desired angle, and thus the tablets may be combined to present the type solids and many common objects of similar forms.

The tablets are light, noiseless, durable, and so inexpensive that each pupil may have a set. They are the best size for free-hand drawing, being two and one-half times the size of the models usually intended for individual use. They are large enough to use for tracing in design and color work. In the study of working drawings, they furnish each pupil an extended range of subjects so that copying is unnecessary.

The slate can rarely be used the first primary year for the testing of the perspective appearance of objects, as the pupils are not old enough to hold it and compare the drawing with the object.

Before the slate is used for the testing of the perspective appearance of form, a sphere, cylindrical pail, an apple, or other simple large object, may be truthfully represented by many pupils in the first primary grade, if they have not studied the actual facts of solids in the mechanical way which prevents conceptions of their appearances. Even the first year pupils should draw occasionally from simple large objects. The drawings should be upon paper and should be large and entirely free-hand. An occasional exercise of this kind will show the capacity for seeing which has been gained, and will prove the value of study upon the slate from the geometric forms.

In the grammar grades and the high school, models can be provided by the pupils, who may bring vases, boxes, bags, baskets, and all kinds of articles which they may wish to draw; but these objects should not be drawn in the lower grades, except occasionally to test the capacity of the pupils.

When rightly taught, interest in the subject of drawing will not depend upon the object of the lesson or upon the making of drawings, which may falsely cause the pupils to think that they are really doing something valuable. The greatest interest will be aroused by the work which causes each pupil to think for himself all the time, and to discover for himself the truths of Nature. This is necessary when pupils draw from the geometric objects, using the slate to correct their drawings, and to point out the inaccuracies of their reasoning; and when, after a time, they become able to make a drawing which does "fit" the first time, they are often unable to restrain their enthusiasm, and greater interest in the subject could be desired by no one.

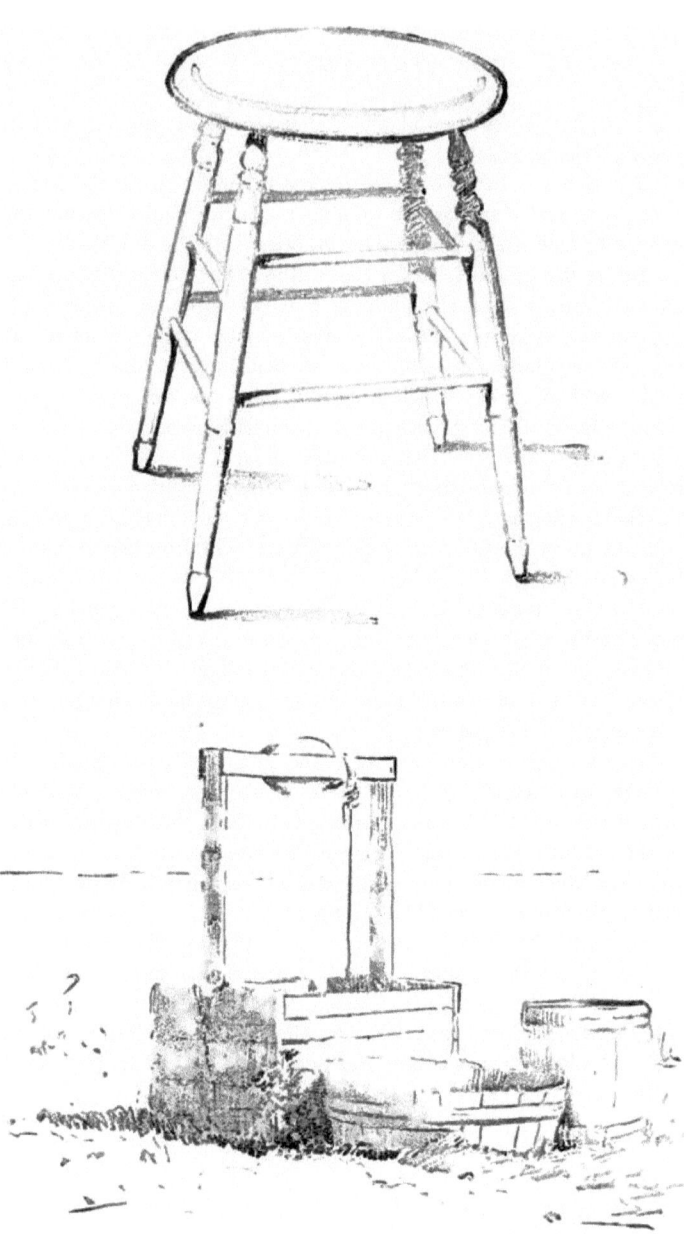

From the National Drawing Books.

room. The expense and nature of the materials would prevent school use, even if there were no other reasons why the system should not be used.

The difficulty of using brush and color or ink in tracing upon glass, and the clumsiness of the wire screen and chalk, have rendered their use, particularly with young pupils, simply an interesting experiment.

To make practical use of the principle, a pencil which will draw freely upon the glass must be used. With such a pencil the glass may take the place of paper, and the principle enables even the young child to test his drawing quickly and surely. This pencil must be one which will draw a fine line and be tough enough not to break easily. After long study and experiment, a pencil has been made which is tough and durable, and which marks as readily upon the glass as upon paper.

If, instead of tracing, the appearance of an object is sketched by eye upon the slate, the drawing may be tested, when it is thought correct, by holding the glass in front of the object and moving it back and forth until the lines of the drawing appear to cover those of the object. If a sheet of white paper is placed behind the glass, the drawing will appear as if on the paper, and there is no difference, so far as its making is concerned, between the use of paper and the transparent glass slate. When the drawing is completed, the difference between the use of the slate and the paper appears. The best teacher is often unable to make the pupil see that his drawing on paper is incorrect ; while the errors of the drawing upon the slate are shown when it is held in front of the object. The pupil is then his own teacher.

The slate should not be used for tracing the appearance — not that Madame Cavé's system has not accomplished much good, but that when used in this way, the result is less satisfactory than when the drawing is made by eye alone, as upon a sheet of paper.

It is not meant that tracing of beautiful forms may not help to realize their beauty, and that work of this nature once in a while may not be profitable, but that object drawing should be by eye alone.

We learn by experience. We may watch an artist draw and paint for a long time, and, if we have never tried to draw or paint, receive little benefit. The teacher who draws much for the student is not teaching. The student who copies is not drawing in its true sense.

We must depend upon the eye for all good results. We train the eye when we discover its mistakes. If a person does not discover that the circle seen obliquely appears an ellipse, he will see it a circle all his life. He will always see the local colors of objects unless he sometimes discovers that something which he did not recognize, appeared very different from its actual color. The only way to train the eye is to depend upon it, and for this reason the student should always draw what is before him without measuring or testing in any way. He should draw upon the slate when the flap is behind it, and should remove the flap to test the drawing only when, after careful observation, he thinks it is what he sees.

The limit to the age when this slate may be used is determined by the ability of the pupil to hold it for testing the drawing at about right angles to the direction in which the object is seen. Some very young pupils will do this readily, and some older ones will have much trouble. One of the greatest difficulties that I have found during my teaching in art schools is, that students measure with the pencil tipped away from them ten or twenty degrees or more, and make drawings to agree with the incorrect measurements thus resulting, even when they can see proportions correctly. They apparently prefer to depend upon these false tests rather than to take the trouble to use their eyes. Of course nothing can prevent or excuse careless-ness, and all that is claimed for the slate is that it may be of great assistance when rightly used.

For use outside the public schools, the student may begin with a large sheet of paper or a circular or square card placed on the floor or on the table. He may then take a box or other common object. It will be seen that the subject studied must be, if small, quite near the eye : thus the student who draws at home has the advantage of the student in the classroom, for he has the choice of all the objects in the room, and may work with them near or distant, according to their sizes.

It will be well always to make the drawing on the slate as large as possible and yet have it cover the object when the slate is held at arm's length.

The slate should not be used for beginners when the models are small and at a distance.

Whatever the size of the models, they should be so near that the drawing which will cover them will be not less than about two inches high. The limit to size will vary with the subject of the lesson, but the drawing must be large enough to admit of comparison. If it is impossible to place the model near enough so that the drawing upon the slate, when made the desired size, will appear to coincide with the object, the directions of its lines may be tested by moving the slate so that the lines may cover those of the object, one at a time. But for the young pupil to get the best results from the work, the models must be placed so that a drawing of fair size can be held in such a way as to appear to coincide with the object.

The slate may be used to test the accuracy of a drawing on paper by tracing this drawing onto the slate, and then holding it before the object in the usual manner.

The slate at once introduces in the most forcible way the subject of appearances entirely separate from and in contradiction to the facts. After a little study upon it, many of the pupils are found to draw at first trial fairly well by eye, and it will be well to discard the slate, at least part of the time, or to use it as a test in the way just explained.

The reason why free-hand drawing has always been so difficult to teach is that no sure way of awakening the first correct impression of the appearance of the form has been given the student. When this impression has been received and appreciated, the rest is easy and consists simply in practice.

The objection of some that the slate may be used to trace the appearance, and that it is thus simply a mechanical means of making a drawing, will apply when teachers allow or advise pupils to work in this way. When, however, they are told how to use the slate properly, there will be few who will not find such use more interesting than the tracing of the form, and those who disobey and trace will even then obtain a better idea of the apparent form than they would without the slate.

Tracing is, however, quite impossible in any except the first lessons from objects placed upon the desks, or so that the slate may rest upon the desk or other support. The slate cannot be held steadily by the hand, and this is the effective safeguard against its improper use. When a drawing has been made upon the slate, it may be held with both hands steadily enough so that it may be compared with the object, and its proportions and masses tested ; but the tracing of more than a line or two of the distant object will be impossible until the slate is held and a sight fixed for the eye ; and such aids to mechanical work should not be given the pupil.

In the drawings of groups of models it will be difficult to hold the slate so as to compare the smallest details. The masses, and the directions of all important lines can, however, be seen, and the pupil who trains his eye to give these correctly will have little trouble with the minor points. As the size of the subject and the number of its parts increase, so does the difficulty of holding the slate so that it may give more than the principal masses ; therefore the pupil who does not understand that the slate is not given as a means for tracing will be disappointed in its use.

A tracing of a large subject which is near, or any extended subject such as an interior, becomes a plane perspective drawing, which always distorts large parts of what it represents. It is impossible to make a tracing upon a slate placed near the eye, of any extended subject which shall represent the different parts of the extended subject just as they appear. In order to represent such subjects with the best success, the draughtsman must have made a careful study of the theory of appearances and the distortions of plane perspective. He cannot avoid error by mechanical means, such as tracing, or the use of photographs, which are frequently the most distorted representations it is possible to make. The avoidance of some distortion of detail in a drawing representing a wide field of view is impossible ; but this is a question of theory which is considered in Chapter VII.

The special pencil required for use upon the slate is called the Cross Pencil. It is sold by Ginn & Co. and marks as readily upon glass, china, or any polished surface, as upon paper.

The pencils are of an oily nature and should not be placed near a radiator as they will become too soft for use. If pencils should soften by heat they will harden when placed in a cool place. To give the best results the pencil, slate, and air should be at about the same temperature.

CHAPTER IV.

SPECIAL DIRECTIONS FOR TEACHERS.

DRAWING ON THE SLATE.

THE teacher who does not understand how to draw, or how to use the glass slate, must prepare for her work by drawing upon the slate just as her pupils do. A short time spent in this study will enable her to draw well enough to give good advice and criticism to her pupils.

The teacher who understands how to draw and how to use the slate, will require little instruction in the details of her work; and she will obtain the best results by depending upon her own judgment instead of upon directions given by those who have no knowledge of her pupils and of their varying needs.

It is impossible to carry out with different classes lengthy and detailed directions, even if they have been successfully followed in special cases. The directions given here are to be considered as suggestions for the experiments which may show teachers the best ways of handling the subject in their own classrooms.

In the primary grades the slate may be placed flat upon the desk during the work in drawing; but as soon as possible it should be held in the left hand, at right angles to the direction in which it is seen; since when flat upon the desk the surface of the slate is generally foreshortened and pupils cannot see the real proportions of their drawings.

The pencil should be as long as possible. It should be held lightly in the fingers, near the middle or at the unsharpened end, for all except the final accenting of the sketch and the drawing of lines at one touch, for which work it must be held nearer the point and more firmly.

The first practice should be in free arm movements and should aim to make the pupils work freely by first suggesting the whole drawing in light touches, and then adding others until the desired effect is obtained by a gradual development or growth of the parts, in which every line and touch helps every other.

The point most necessary for the pupils to understand is that they cannot expect to draw correctly at first touch, and that it is useless to spend unnecessary time upon lines which must be changed. Of course, practice of free arm movements will enable an approximate straight line or regular curve, as the circle or ellipse, to be drawn with one movement. The power to do this is desirable, but principally because it will enable pupils to obtain correct drawings, after making a comparatively small number of changes in the lines first suggested.

Free arm movements may be practised in the air, upon the slate, or upon paper, and should be repeated frequently. Pupils should be encouraged to spend any spare moments, whether of the drawing hour or other period, in this way.

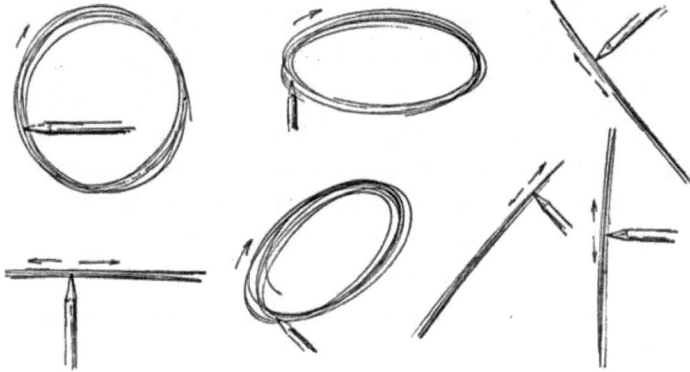

In this practice the motion should be perfectly free and of the whole arm from the shoulder. The lines should be gone over repeatedly with a rapid, continuous motion. In circles and ellipses the motion should be from left to right. In straight lines the pencil should be on the slate or paper all the time, and the lines drawn in both directions.

The printed copies for use in the lower grades are to be so placed on the model support at the back of the desk as to be at right angles to the direction in which they are seen.

The first copies are to be full size, and are to be made by eye without any measurements. They are to be tested by folding the flap back and holding the slate so that the drawing covers the copy. If the drawing is the same size as the copy and is correct, the two will appear to coincide; if incorrect or not the right size, the pupils will at once see what changes to make. These may be made without erasing, unless it is necessary in order that the pupils may see the drawing and the copy at the same time.

.When testing these full-size drawings, the slate must be held against the printed copy, with its long edges horizontal, that is, parallel to those of the book. The book must not be taken from the model support and held behind the slate.

When drawing from the printed lines the pupils should endeavor to give their lengths, positions, and relations, and also to divide them as the copies are divided. In these lessons special care must be taken, when testing, to have the slate held with its edges parallel to those of the book.

The square, circle, and any regular polygon drawn from the copy may be tested, if drawn smaller or larger than full size, by holding the slate so that the drawing and the copy are concentric.

If the pupils are able to close one eye when testing the drawings of copies, tablets, or solids which are smaller than full size, they may be made to appear to coincide with the copy or the object drawn, by holding the slate nearer the eye than the copy or object. As soon as possible this way of testing should be explained and used exclusively.

When able to draw the forms of the simple copies, the pupils may draw from large tablets placed upon the model support so as to appear their real shapes. The drawings may be tested as were those from the printed cards.

The circle and square should be drawn first, and repeatedly, and then the other tablets. The polygons should be placed in many different positions so that their edges may have all possible relations to the desk. These tablets should be drawn until the pupils can represent their real shapes correctly.

When drawing these forms, practice in comparing distances may be given by placing points for the centres of the figures. When placed, the positions of the points should be tested.

Drawings made on paper may be tested by tracing them upon the slate and then by holding the slate and comparing in the usual manner. Drawings from copies, tablets, or solids may be made and tested in this way. It is, however, not as generally satisfactory as the direct use of the slate.

The drawings should be made without placing points for the ends of lines and the corners of figures, except when the work is intended to be dictation. There should be one method for all the work, and it should be artistic instead of mechanical. If pupils begin by placing points it will be difficult for them to change and consider the masses (the whole) in later work.

FORESHORTENING.

The circular or square tablet may be placed horizontally at the back of the desk for the first lesson involving foreshortening. No study of theory or explanation of principles is necessary or advisable. Let the pupils arrange and draw the tablets, and then test by holding the slates as they have held them when drawing from the copies and the cards when not foreshortened. After a few experiments they will understand that the tablets do not appear their real shapes, and they will be interested to study other forms in the same way.

Pupils who begin the use of the slate by drawing from the printed copies will have little difficulty in using it to test the drawings of foreshortened forms. Any pupil who is unable to hold the slate to test perspective drawings will be assisted by placing a piece of paper about ⅛" in diameter upon the desk and marking a point upon the slate. He will readily hold the slate so that the point appears to cover the paper.

After this he may place a stick upon the desk, and draw upon the slate a line shorter than the stick. By holding the slate in front of the stick, and changing the distance of the slate and its angle with the desk, the line may be made to appear to coincide with the stick ; and in the same way it may be made to appear to cover any line whatever in the room. These experiments will help the pupils to understand that a correct picture of any tablet or object must appear, in every part, to coincide with the corresponding part of the object.

The problem may be simplified for young pupils by having the nearest point or edge of the tablet touch the slate, and the slate rest upon the desk, so as to be held steadily for the test. In order that the tablets touch the slate, they must be raised from the desk by a book or other object. When thus arranged, the slate is to be placed upon the desk and against the tablet, and held by the left hand at right angles to the direction in which the tablet is seen; while with the pencil held in the right hand the angle or edge of the tablet on the slate is traced. The slate is then to be taken up and the drawing completed by eye, above its lowest point or line traced on the slate. To test the drawing, the slate is placed in the position it had when the point or edge of the tablet on the slate was traced.

When the tablet is placed upon a small object, the slate may be supported as an easel by opening it at an angle with the flap, and resting the two parts on the desk as illustrated. This enables the pupil to give his entire attention to the comparison of the drawing and the object.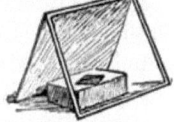

In all this work, when the test is applied, the eye should be in the same position it had when the drawing was made. These first experiments give, however, simply an idea of perspective, and this will be gained if the positions are not exactly the same.

When pupils are allowed to begin in this way, they should, as quickly as possible after this method, be taught to hold the slate at arm's length, and nearer the eye than the object, in order that they may make drawings which are more pleasing than those which will result from the eye being near the object and some distance above it.

Few pupils who have drawn from the printed copies and the tablets placed to appear their real shapes, will have much trouble in using the slate properly in work involving foreshortening. Tracing to a greater extent than that indicated above should not be allowed, for many of the pupils will not think of tracing if it is not explained, and thus they will not be tempted to avoid work by tracing instead of drawing.

Having drawn from the circular and square tablets, the pupils may be led to see that these may appear straight lines, or figures of any width up to their actual width. To illustrate this fact in the simplest way, cut a circular piece of paper with a projecting piece at one side, and hold the circle against the back of the slate while tracing its real shape. Then swing the circle back and observe its appearance when it is at different angles to the slate. This experiment with the circle, a similar one with the square (see Lesson I., page 56), and, if desired, with the triangle, or other forms, may be made and understood by young pupils. Theories and rules, however, should not be stated until the pupils have had more experience.

In arranging tablets and other objects for study, no care should be taken to obtain definite angles as 60°, 45°, or 30°, etc. The simplest foreshortened position of the rectangle is when two edges appear horizontal. When the illustrations represent this position, all the tablets of the class should be so placed; but when the illustrations show tablets at angles, the angles are not specified and are immaterial, and each pupil's tablet may be in a different position.

When able to represent single tablets, two may be combined and placed in different positions, as illustrated in the "Outlines of Lessons."

If the slates are used accurately enough to give the convergence seen in the vertical edges, when drawing tablets and single objects, there is no reason why this convergence should not be represented until the pupils are older, and the work more advanced, when they may be told that it is the custom to omit this convergence and represent vertical edges by vertical lines.

After drawing from two tablets combined, several tablets may be arranged in the form of the type solids, or of common objects based upon them. The interior and the exterior of the solid prism forms should be studied, by combining the tablets to present these appearances.

To obtain the cube, for free-hand purposes, it is necessary to combine only two or three square tablets; and no more tablets should be used for any form than are necessary to give the visible surfaces for the required position of the object.

The prism forms are best represented, for free-hand purposes, by tablets representing the bases, and connected by a rod which represents the axis of the prism. Both ends of the prism are thus visible at the same time.

For the first few years all tablets and combinations of tablets should be placed at the middle of the back of the desk, for the desk line behind the tablets will then appear horizontal and assist the pupils to correct their work. If the tablets are placed at the corner of the desk, the desk line will appear inclined and the problem is much more difficult.

The desk line (called table line) should not be represented in the first work, for it is thought of as horizontal, and when in later work it does not appear horizontal, the pupils will, if in the habit of representing it by a horizontal line, be prevented from seeing correctly the directions of the lines of the object. In the upper grades, and after having drawn from objects at a distance and not directly in front of the pupils (when referred to the desk or the walls of the room), the table line or edge of the shelf supporting the objects may be represented, but always as an inclined line when its ends or points in it on each side, equally distant from the group, are unequally distant from the eye. The custom of drawing a horizontal line to represent this edge, when it seldom appears horizontal, is one of the many evil results of the teaching which assumes that drawing can be understood and taught by mental processes only.

In some cities an adjustable model-support is used, which is attached at the corner of the desk, and is valuable as it gives any desired elevation to the object. When this is used in the lower grades, its edges should not be parallel to those of the desk. The edges should be so placed that the ends of the nearer edge are equally distant from the pupil's eyes. In the upper grades, they should be placed in various positions and their lines represented in every drawing.

After the pupils are able to draw and test with ease the tablets and combinations of tablets placed on their own desks, they should draw from objects farther away. Drawings on the slate ought never to be less than about two or three inches long, according to the subject studied. The drawing which will appear to cover a distant object, will be much too small to be satisfactory unless the object is quite large. All drawings on the slate or on paper should be of fair size, and, as large drawings cannot be made to appear to cover the object, it is necessary to find some new way to test their proportions. The use of the pencil to obtain the proportions of objects is explained in Chapter V, and also in the "Grammar Outline of Lessons," and, after the slate, is the method of most value to the pupils.

Drawings which are too large to appear to coincide with the object may be tested by holding the slate so that, one at a time, the different points of the drawing may appear to cover the corresponding points of the object. In this way the directions of all the lines meeting at a point may be tested, and if the directions are correct throughout the drawing, the proportions must be also.

In the upper grades memory drawings of the cube, cylinder, and other type forms may be made on the slate. These may be tested by placing the object at any level and angle such that the drawing on the slate may be made to appear to coincide with the object. When a memory drawing represents a possible appearance of any object, a few experiments will give the position of the object in which the drawing will appear to coincide with it.

The chief value of the slate consists in the instant and certain test of proportions given by its use. Many pupils who use the slate through the lower grades will, when in the upper grades, have little need for it or other means of testing, as they will be able to depend upon their eyes; and all pupils of the upper grammar grades will find the best use of the slate to be in the rapid sketching, by eye entirely, of large simple objects whose proportions may be tested by holding the sketch upon the slate to cover the object, in the usual manner.

Pupils must expect to make sketches, and not finished drawings, upon the slate. Having used the slate, they will understand what a sketch is, and, more important, will be able to work in a sketchy and artistic manner.

The slate may be used for reviews of the facts of form, for the free-hand working drawings made in studying principles preliminary to the instrumental drawings, and for all work in drawing which is not intended to be kept to show the capacity of the students.

The fact that the work done upon the slate is not kept, is beneficial; for most unsatisfactory results are due to the instruction commonly given, by which pupils are assisted to perform a certain amount of work, all of which is kept as if it were valuable.

The objection of some to the use of the slate is that the supervisor cannot see all the work done by the pupils. This is not considered important, for pupils cannot draw without study, and if the practice work is not done, the drawings on paper or in the book will show it, and the supervisor can at any time ask that all the drawings be made on paper, if for any reason he desires to see them.

When the air is very damp and the slate is cold, the moisture will condense upon it, and the pencil will not work until the slate has been rubbed with a dry cloth or warmed. There are in a school year but few days when this trouble will occur, and it is readily remedied as explained above, or avoided by drawing on paper.

The slate should be cleaned at the end of each lesson, as the lines are more readily removed at this time than at any later period. A dry woolen cloth with a rough surface should be used for erasing. Albatross cloth or nun's veiling is the best.

DRAWING ON PAPER.

When books are not used, pupils should draw upon blocks or upon sheets of paper fastened to small drawing boards, so that the paper, during all except the finishing or accenting of the drawing, may be held at right angles to the direction in which it is seen. *This is especially important, and in all free-hand drawing the slate, book, or block should be held at right angles to the direction in which it is seen.*

Drawings upon separate sheets of paper should be numbered and dated, and arranged in order in large envelopes kept for this purpose by the pupils.

The drawing books should be fastened to cardboard or other backs, in order that they may be used as blocks. The book may be placed upon the model support, which is changed into a desk easel by extending the base, or held in the hand while the first sketching is done; but it may be placed flat upon the desk when the drawing is ready for accenting.

When copies from the book are to be drawn on the slate, the book should be supported by the cardboard back and placed upon the model support.

For the upper grades the pupils should be asked to make drawings from outdoor subjects of a simple nature, and from any objects, found at home or elsewhere, which interest them. A cheap sketch book is the best means of interesting the pupils and of keeping the drawings. These books may be criticised by the teacher occasionally.

A few moments' talk once in a while upon the pictures of the magazines will interest and instruct the pupils. Such drawings should be cut out and fastened upon the walls.

The reproductions of artists' and old masters' drawings, given in each drawing book, are valuable, as they furnish each pupil the best inspiration for individual work, even when they are drawing the type forms in outline; and they give the pupils of the upper grades the best information of the way in which the drawings they desire to make at home should be handled.

These reproductions are not intended as copies, but pupils who work at home and out-of-doors will be helped by copying a drawing once in a while, after having attempted original drawings in the same style of handling. This copying should not be done during the drawing period.

When working from foliage, flowers, fruits, or vegetables, the aim should be for artistic, and not for structural or botanical drawings. Drawings which give all the minute veins and details of these subjects may be made for the study of botany, but the drawing hour should be devoted to artistic rendering, to the study of the masses and the effect, and not to details of growth which are unimportant artistically.

Details of foliage and vegetable growths may be studied in about the following order, though this is unimportant if too difficult work is not given.

Single, large, simple leaves placed so their real shapes are seen.

Vegetables and fruit.

Single, large leaves when foreshortened.

Face views of flowers.

Side views of flowers.

Sprays of foliage placed so the leaves appear their real shapes.

Sprays of foliage placed in any natural position.

Sprays of foliage and flowers in any natural position.

Foliage and flowers, as in potted plants.

Sprays of foliage may be placed in bottles filled with water or with wet sand. The sand will hold them firmly in position.

Plants with simple, large leaves, such as the geranium, calla lily, begonia, primrose, gloxinia, cowslip, jack-in-the-pulpit, and rubber plant, may be placed on boards across the aisles and drawn by the pupils of the eighth grade.

BLACKBOARD DRAWING.

Pupils who work for a long time upon drawings of uniform size find it very difficult to make larger or smaller drawings; for this reason blackboard drawings should be made occasionally. *These drawings should be of the same nature as the other work.* As few pupils can work on the board at the same time, this work should be done outside the drawing period; and if it is not possible to place objects so that pupils may draw from them, they may draw from memory. The making of "pictures," copying, etc., should not be allowed.

CHAPTER V.

TESTS.

In beginning, the pupil should understand that his drawings are of no value in themselves, but are of use only as they train the eye to see correctly. The eye can be taught, or rather the mind can be made to accept the image of the eye, only by depending upon it: *if the student begins by measuring and testing he will never be able to draw otherwise.* Depending upon measurements is undesirable for many reasons, the most important being that no measurements can be applied which will take the place of correct perception, or begin to equal the trained eye. It is thus important that the student, from the beginning, depend entirely for his first drawing upon his eyes.

The best possible training for all, young or old, is the use of the glass slate.

Without the slate, the readiest way of determining the apparent proportions of an object is by the use of a pencil or any straight, slender rod held at arm's length, so as to appear to cover the dimensions of the object which are to be compared.

Thus, if the top of the pencil, when it is held at right angles to the direction in which the object is seen and so as to appear vertical, is made to cover the top of an object, and the bottom of the object is marked upon the pencil by the thumb nail, the distance thus set off on the pencil measures the apparent height of the object. If the pencil is now revolved to a horizontal position, the apparent height may be compared with the apparent width by holding the pencil so that its end appears to cover the left point of the object. If the width appears the same as the height, the thumb nail will appear to cover the right point of the object. If the width is greater or less than the height, the proportion may be readily observed.

The shorter measurement should always be compared with the longer.

The pencil must be at right angles to the direction in which the object is seen. Nearly all students think the pencil should be parallel to the side of the room or the bench upon which the object rests. This, however, is wholly false, for the position of the object with reference to its surroundings is of no consequence, and must not be considered when the actual appearance of the object is desired. If a cube is to be represented, the student must look at it. The plane which gives its real appearance is perpendicular to the direction in which he looks, and when measuring, the pencil must always be held in this position. When thus held, its ends are the same distance from the eye, and the pencil is not vertical when the student looks at an object above or below the level of the eye.[1]

A good plan is to find some position in the fingers in which the

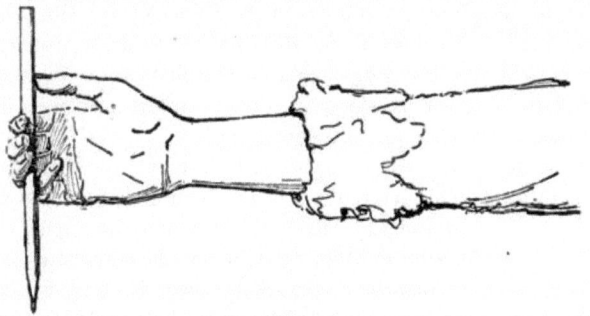

FIG. 12.

pencil is perpendicular to the arm, which, when outstretched, brings the pencil into practically the correct position. See Fig. 12.

It is important that this use of the pencil shall determine simply the proportion of the drawing and not its actual size. The measurements on the pencil should not be transferred to the paper; for the eye and hand are generally in different positions when the various measurements are taken, and if they are transferred to the paper the drawing resulting will be incorrect in proportion. Not only this, but the drawing will be limited in size and will often be too small.

The great difficulty in the use of the pencil for measuring is that it is not held properly, — at right angles to the direction in which the

[1] To be exact, the part of the pencil which includes the measurement should be at right angles to the direction in which the pupil sees the object, but practically such fine results cannot be obtained and are unnecessary.

object is seen. Even students in art schools, after months of study, are frequently seen measuring with the pencil foreshortened to the extent of 20 or 30 degrees. This may be avoided by measuring from the unsharpened end of the pencil instead of from the sharpened end; for when the pencil is held so that the flat end appears a straight line, it must be about at right angles to the direction in which the object is seen.

A much better device, especially for young pupils, is a rod about as long as a pencil, its outer surface black, with the two ends cut squarely and of the natural color of the wood. When this measuring rod is held so that neither light end is seen, it is in the proper position for measuring; but if one of the white ends is visible, the rod is at an angle. A substitute for this special rod is an unsharpened pencil. This simple device should enable all to measure properly, and will be of great assistance to those teachers who now find it impossible to have the pencil properly held.

The same result may be obtained by bending a hairpin about a large knitting needle, as shown in Fig. 13. One end of the hairpin, *A*,

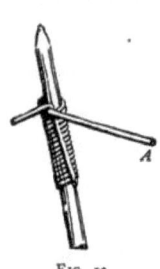

projects for about an inch at right angles to the needle and forms a sight, and the other, after passing around the needle several times, is brought back and projects a short distance at right angles to the first end. The longer end serves to place the needle at right angles to the line of vision, for when only the end of the sight is seen, the needle must be properly placed. The wire should press the needle enough to stay in position upon it. It may be

FIG. 13.

moved so that the measurement is included between the end of the needle and the short projecting end of the wire. When the needle is turned for comparison, the second measurement may be taken by the thumb nail, and the proportions may then be determined at leisure; this is the only advantage of this device over the straight rod with ends at right angles to the rod, and the simpler rod will be all that is necessary for most students.

The proportions of any object may also be accurately measured by the simple object illustrated in Fig. 14. It consists of two parts: first, a card which has a long rectangular opening, and second, a sliding part made by folding and gluing together around the card a piece of paper which serves as a shutter, and which may be moved to give any proportion to the opening cut in the card. By holding the card so that the opening measures the height of an object, and moving the shutter until the width is covered, the two dimensions may be correctly obtained, and may be compared at leisure. To facilitate comparison, one vertical and one horizontal edge of the card may have set off upon them equal spaces as ⅛″, ¼″, or ½″, according to the size of the opening.

This card will also be valuable in determining the arrangement of the drawing upon the paper. It serves as a frame to the subject, and may be shifted until the best position of the sketch upon the paper is determined.

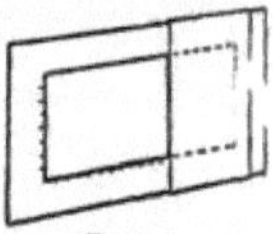

When proportions are compared, the distance of the needle or pencil from the eye must be the same. The distance is so apt to vary that unless each comparison is made several times with the same result, there is little chance that measurements will be correct. It is useless to think that tests not carefully taken are worth the time given them. It is much better to take the one proportion of height and width carefully, than to spend the time necessary to do this on half a dozen measurements which are sure to contradict, and do more harm than good.

Fig. 14.

It is impossible to compare accurately a short distance, with one many times greater. If the height is equal to or is nearly one-half or one-third of the width, care will so determine it; but with every new position of the hand in moving a short distance over a long, inaccuracy arises, and it is well to avoid such comparisons, for they are not only not to be depended upon but are unnecessary.

The inaccuracy is produced by inability to hold the pencil at exactly the right place, and also by the change in the distance of the pencil which every movement away from the first position occasions.

This movement may be realized by tying a thread to the pencil and measuring its distance from the eye by holding the thread with the left hand against the brow. If the arm is dropped for the measurement of a near object and the string is tight, it will loosen when the arm is raised, and in the same way it will change for horizontal movement. The only way in which exact measurements of an extended subject can be taken is by the use of such a measuring-thread attached to the measuring rod. We wish to simplify the subject as much as possible. If reasonable care is exercised, the variation in the distance of the pencil, when used without a measuring-thread, may be made so slight as to be unimportant in the drawing of small objects.

When possible, all comparisons should be made by swinging the pencil from a vertical into a horizontal position by motion of the

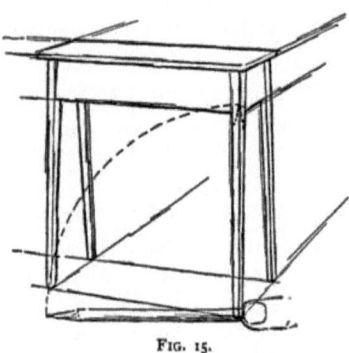

FIG. 15.

whole arm from the shoulder, avoiding change · in distance by revolving the pencil about one end of the first measurement. Thus, if the height and width of a table are to be compared, instead of measuring the width along the top and dropping the hand to compare the width with the height, or measuring the height and then lifting the hand to compare with the width, make the comparison by taking the width along the top and swinging the pencil down about the thumb; or by taking the width at the bottom and swinging the pencil up about the thumb, as in Fig. 15. Measuring in this way will assist greatly to correct results.

The above are the direct tests for proportion, and if carefully taken should give the correct mass of the drawing; but for the directions of lines other tests are better.

It is natural to compare directions with vertical and horizontal lines. A horizontal line whose ends are equidistant from the eye appears horizontal, and is represented by a horizontal line. A vertical line appears vertical, and is always represented by a vertical line. If a ruler is held horizontal, with its ends equally distant from the eye, it illustrates the appearance represented by a horizontal line in the drawing. By looking over the ruler thus held, the apparent directions of lines of the object may be compared with the horizontal.

A' thread with a weight attached serves as a plumb-line. By holding the plumb-line in front of the object, the lines of the object may be compared with the vertical. The thread may also be used, and is often better than the ruler or pencil, for the horizontal line, as it hides none of the object. Care must always be taken to hold the thread perpendicular to a line from the eye to the object. This position is easiest obtained by directly facing the group, extending the arms equally, and holding in each hand one end of a piece of thread about two feet long.

More care must be exercised to have the thread horizontal. This position can be obtained by looking only at the thread until it is levelled, when the student may look beyond it at the group. If there are horizontal lines in the subject which are parallel to the picture plane they will appear horizontal and will place the thread correctly; but if the horizontal lines of the subject are not thus situated, they will not appear horizontal, and will cause the thread to seem horizontal when it is inclined.

It may seem that unnecessary space has been given to these directions, but it has been found almost impossible to make many students understand the matter and hold the thread correctly, even after repeated explanations and illustrations. Some, after months of study, are found holding the thread or pencil at an angle of from ten to thirty degrees away from the correct position, and it is thought that no explanation can be too careful. The problem is so simple that any student who wishes to succeed should have no difficulty; he may be sure that he will never learn to draw until he is able to discover his mistakes, and as the use of the thread is a most important test, it should be correctly applied.

Any object, as the cube, Fig. 16 having been drawn, may be tested by

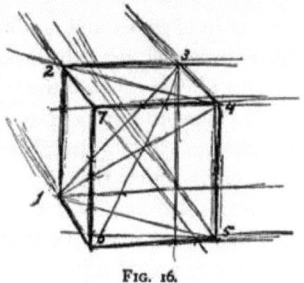

FIG. 16.

the thread as follows: Hold the thread horizontally to cover point 5, and note its apparent intersection with the edges 1–6 and 6–7. Hold the thread vertically in front of point 3, and see where it intersects

5–6. Hold it in front of 6–7, and notice its intersection with 2–3. Hold the thread to cover 1 and 5, also 2 and 4, and compare its direction with a horizontal line. Continue the edge 2–7 to intersect 5–6, and 4–7 to intersect 2–1. Cover any opposite points, as 1 and 3, 3 and 6, 4 and 1, etc., and notice where the thread appears to intersect the edges between.

This use of the thread is simply a more exact method of discovering angles than drawing lines in the air, the method explained on p. 5. When the eye is trained, the first, which is of course the simpler, is all that is needed. Most students will find the use of the thread necessary. The thread gives a fine line which can be made to exactly cover the edges of the object, and its intersections with the edges can be seen much more readily than those of a line formed by a pencil or rule, which hides considerable of the object. If these tests with the thread are applied, they cannot fail to discover every error of importance.

The thread should not be used to measure the proportions of objects.

A last test may be applied by holding two pencils together at right angles to the direction in which the object is seen, and separating them until one covers 3–4, and the other covers 1–6. If great care is taken, the directions of these lines with reference to each other may be seen, and the drawing tested by continuing these lines in the drawing.

The apparent angle between two lines may be measured by folding a strip of paper and holding it so that each part appears to coincide with one of the two lines. This test is easiest applied by the use of a hinged rule or straight-edge of two parts.

The two tests just explained cannot be recommended for pupils, since there are two straight-edges to be held at right angles to the direction in which the object is seen. It is so difficult to do this that those who can hold the rules correctly may depend upon their eyes, and get the drawing better without these tests than with them.

Another way of testing the direction of a line is to hold a straight edge upon the line of the drawing so that it will project beyond the board, and then lift the board and straight edge into the position of the picture plane, when the straight edge appears to coincide with the edge of the object if the direction of the line in the drawing is correct.

I have dwelt thus carefully upon these tests in the hope that the student may realize their importance, for he will learn to draw correctly only through his own efforts, gaining with each discovery of error. He can never become a draughtsman as long as he depends upon a teacher for corrections. Let him carry his drawing so far that a thorough application of all the tests explained will show no error; then, as it is simply a question of exactness to be determined by the eye, if the trained eye of the teacher discovers mistakes so slight that the student cannot rightly be expected to determine them, these may be pointed out. As the chief benefit results from what the student himself sees and does, he will be much better off without a teacher than with one who does his work for him.

The advanced art student should use few tests, and should not require the mechanical aids which have been explained. These different ways of testing have been given, because the teacher should understand them all. They should not, however, be explained to the pupils, at least not at once, or following one another closely; some of them are not suitable for pupils to attempt, and should not be explained. The pupil who begins with the slate, and later uses the measuring rod and the thread, will not require other tests, nor even these, through the entire course. When correcting pupils' drawings, the teacher may sometimes find other tests than the slate valuable and convenient. At such times, ways of testing, such as the use of the straight edge (p. 48), may be explained to advanced pupils, but at first the glass slate, and later the thread and measuring rod, should be depended upon.

Some artists say that students should use no test but their eyes, and that even the pencil for measuring proportions, or the thread for directions and intersections, are means which are too mechanical, and which should be avoided. They say that the pupil should be led to "feel" errors in his drawing.

As a rule, those who are strongest in the expression of such ideas, if teachers, are teachers of advanced students. It is thought that any one who has had much experience with pupils who have never learned to draw will say that feeling must generally come after some ability to see has been acquired ; and that to teach them to see correctly is a most difficult problem in which the teacher's eyes cannot serve the pupil. This problem can only be solved by means which prove to the student the falsity of the work, which, until the tests are applied, seems perfect to him.

As the pencil is often held carelessly, its use by students who have had some training frequently does them more harm than good ; especially when they measure before drawing, for they make drawings to agree with incorrect measurements, when, if they would use their eyes, they would see the proportions more correctly.

Any means which are used to take the place of the eyes, or any tests which are applied before drawing, must harm the student, for they make it difficult for him to use his eyes, and weaken him in proportion as he studies in this mechanical way. But tests that are applied after the student has carried his drawing as far as he can without testing, are not mechanical so far as results are concerned, and, if they show the drawing which was thought correct to be incorrect, they must be educational and valuable. The only way to produce successful results is to make the student independent, and, as far as possible, able to test the accuracy of his work, when at the point where without the tests he can do no more. In form he can do this quite perfectly, and, if he applies tests only after the drawing has been carried as far as possible without them, he will advance rapidly.

In light and shade the use of a lens of about fifteen inches' focus to blur the effect, is a mechanical aid which enables the student to believe his own eyes, and see, for instance, that a black vase may appear lighter than a gray cast, when without the glass he would fail to see it, even after half an hour's talk by the teacher. This glass will also prove a valuable aid in color study. It may be mechanical, but it will enable the student to see effects truly and finally to "feel" the sentiment in Nature. It will do this much more quickly than the teacher, who is unable to prove himself right to the student who fails to see color or values as he does.

The right use of tests, such as the slate, pencil, thread, and blur glass, quickly renders the use of all tests unnecessary by training the eye to see correctly. For instance, the use of the blur glass for a very short time will enable the student to realize what the masses are, and to see simply without mechanical aid — to see, in fact, much better than is possible with such help; for the eye can focus to give any desired amount of detail.

If the artist who has forgotten his first struggles in drawing and who wishes students to be taught to feel, will take a class of average pupils and try to give them this power without the assistance of tests applied by the students, he will be more fortunate than most artists who teach, if he does not decide that many of the class have mistaken their vocations. If he has not the privilege of telling them so, or if he fails to make them agree with him, and they still persist in producing work which is completely devoid, not only of sentiment, but also of all vestige of even mechanical truth, the chances are that he will be very glad to give them simple aids to assist them to see, and will, after a short experience, decide that these aids are not only necessary but wise.

While speaking of artists, I wish to refer to the criticisms sometimes made upon the cuts and sketches of many of the drawing-books for students' use. As a rule, these drawings are mechanical and hard when they might be more artistic ; but some criticism is calculated to give the student the idea that artists' sketches do not give the exact geometrical appearance, and that therefore it is useless for the art pupil to draw a perfect line, for instance, an ellipse in the representation of a circle seen obliquely. Such ideas more than anything else are calculated to produce the careless, spotty, and meaningless sketches which are made by students who are searching for handling, technique, and freedom as the all-important ends, when they should be seriously considering how what is before them appears.

Artists who have given their lives to acquiring knowledge may be able to express this knowledge so simply and directly that their work may seem careless to the student : this is no reason for the conclusion that it is carelessly done. The strokes which seem accidental to him, express effects which it has taken the artist perhaps years to see, and which the student cannot see without similar study. The artist's technique is free because by long study he has become able to see truly at a glance, and his only thought in working is the idea to be expressed, and not the handling of the medium.

The pupil, who, after much effort to express the form of a circle which is seen obliquely, can only obtain a line which is as irregular as a brook, ought not to be permitted to think that free handling of his pencil or brush will hide inability to draw, or give a substitute for any of the qualities essential to good work. When he has trained his eye and hand so that they are his servants, it is time to think of handling; but at this time it will not be necessary, for it will come without thought as a result of the knowledge and experience gained by serious study.

The student, then, should not shirk careful drawing nor the most searching study of detail. It is useless for him to think that he can produce a drawing or a picture which has the parts essential to it well studied, if he cannot make a study of a simple group of still life which shall represent all parts of the subject, and every detail, in correct drawing and values. The student who feels that, because all the detail is not always essential, he can omit any before he becomes able to express all by correct drawing and values, if asked so to do, is wasting his time, for he will make drawings which omit the essentials and which are without merit of any kind.

The student who can draw a perfect ellipse easily will have no trouble in representing lines which are not quite circular; and, understanding that a sketch which is artistic must give a sense of atmosphere, he will soon discover that a hard and rigid line is not satisfactory; and, being able to draw freely, his sketches will have the variation of line which is essential. This can never come by avoiding serious study of form and effects.

The student who studies for love of art and not for fashion's sake or for a trade, will discover that popularity is not a sign of merit, and that financial success unfortunately is gained frequently by those who know the least, while serious, honest work is unnoticed by the public, which buys what is simply "pretty" or "clever" or what is the style, without regard to its merit. The serious student must understand that the sketches which were made so rapidly and sell so fast, and for such large prices, are often as devoid of truth as it is possible for them to be. They are conventional in drawing, false in color and values, but attract the eye because they are "sketchy" and interestingly composed. The student should not permit them to influence him to work for such false and cheap results, nor should he be persuaded against his judgment by the popular verdict into accepting this class of work as good and worthy of emulation.

The teacher, then, should not be disturbed by the criticism of superficial art students or critics, but should insist that the students begin to study seriously with only the idea of becoming able to represent truly just what is before them : after this they must depend upon themselves for the artistic feeling which shall decide what is essential, and when changes from the actual appearance will produce a more satisfactory impression than absolute truth of appearance.

This power to feel is only to be gained by depending upon the eye, and teachers should insist that all work be begun before any mechanical tests are applied. At first pupils will not be able to see angles and foreshortening at all correctly, and the tests when applied will show the pupils the errors of their work. But after a little study pupils will be able to see proportions and masses more truly than they can measure them ; and if they are led to think of the apparent widths and heights of the different objects of the group and of each different part of every object, they will be surprised to find that consideration of these proportions will often show the work which their measurements have produced, to be incorrect.

This is due to the fact that pupils are allowed to think of the contour of the object, that is, of the line that they draw to represent it, instead of the space or mass that the line encloses. As long as pupils work in this way they will never feel nor learn to express the sentiment and the artistic qualities of the object before them.

Excellent practice in the observation that leads to successful drawing will be given by placing any simple object before pupils for a few seconds and asking them to observe and remember its appearance and to draw it when the object is taken away. Practice of this nature may be given upon the slate and thus the pupils may test the accuracy of their perception and memory.

CHAPTER VI.

FREE-HAND PERSPECTIVE OR MODEL DRAWING.

THE great differences which exist between the drawings from nature made by artists in a free-hand way, and those obtained by following the rules of scientific perspective cause the perplexing questions which are discussed in Chap. VII. These questions must be considered by the teacher, for even the youngest pupils who discover that parallel retreating lines appear to vanish will wish to know why vertical lines do not appear to vanish, and if so why they are not so represented. In the same way other points will be brought before the teacher, and all teachers should thus understand the subject, at least so as to be able to apply the few rules given in Chap. VII.

Teachers should not, however, discuss the different theories of Chap. VII with young pupils, and all through the grammar school these questions should, as far as possible, be avoided. It will not be difficult to do this, for when· pupils draw from single objects or groups causing small visual angles, the principal difference between what the eye sees and the drawing that the artist makes, is that the artist does not represent the convergence of vertical lines.

Teachers will obtain the best results by beginning the study of free-hand drawing by the use of the slate, which in a short time will make pupils practically familiar with the perspective principles which are valuable to the artist. When pupils have used the slate some time, they may be led to discover and state the principles which govern the appearance of the type forms, and when they can draw correctly, applying the rules to test drawings of single objects and groups causing small visual angles, they may begin to draw interiors and subjects causing large visual angles. But even in this work it is only necessary that drawings be made in accord with the few rules given, and teachers should not expect pupils to generally consider theories upon which experienced instructors and artists are often in doubt; the rules of Chap. VII are all that the pupil requires.

No one ever drew from nature correctly simply from study of theory, and time spent upon theory, whether the free-hand or the scientific, is wasted if some practical ability to draw from nature is not possessed. Pupils who cannot draw approximately correct representations of single simple objects should spend their time in drawing rather than in study of theory ; but those who begin drawing by the use of the slate may quickly understand the most important rules of this chapter, for the slate enables pupils to understand what would otherwise require many months of serious study. Generally the best results will be obtained by giving theory lessons to pupils who have used the slate and can draw fairly well, but teachers may use their judgment upon this point.

Chap. VII shows that the artist makes scientific perspective drawings only when obliged to do so, as such drawings are generally very different from the appearances which objects present to the eye ; and teachers must decide that young pupils should not study scientific perspective, nor any pupils who wish to draw free-hand, until they are able to draw from simple objects correctly and understand model drawing.

Scientific perspective has caused much harm to art, for false representations of prism forms are generally accepted as correct, and the art student who discovers that the subject gives drawings very different from what he sees often wholly neglects perspective, to the great detriment of his work.

Scientific perspective is absolutely necessary to the artist, who often finds that it gives the most satisfactory representation of a geometric subject. It is also valuable to the architect and the illustrator, and the teacher should understand its principles. But whenever it is taught, the fact that its drawings differ from what the eye sees, and are distortions unless seen from the station-point, should be carefully explained.

For most of an artist's work knowledge of model drawing is not only all that he requires, but better than knowledge of scientific perspective. The principles of model drawing are few and simple, and even the young pupil, if he will follow the directions given, will find the free-hand perspective interesting and easy to understand ; for there are no planes, lines, and points to be imagined, and no difficult processes to be understood and carried out. There is no confusion resulting from many technical names and operations. The subject may be presented so that it can be readily understood, and should be studied, as it will be of value to all. .

LESSONS.

The following lessons are to be given in the public schools as indicated in the "Outline of Lessons for Grammar Grades." They are not to be given to pupils who are unable to draw the forms by eye alone with some degree of correctness.

Lesson I. — Foreshortened Planes and Lines.

Cut from paper a circle and a square 4″ in diameter, having projecting pieces as at *A* and *B*. Place the circle upon the back of the

slate and trace its real shape. Then swing the circle back and trace its foreshortened appearance.

Draw the real shape and the foreshortened appearance of the square in the same way, holding the slate vertical, and so that half the square is above and half below the level of the eye.

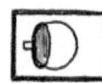

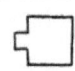

The cards are to be held against the slate by means of the projecting pieces, and they should be revolved so that they are seen edgewise and at different angles.

A square card may be cut so as to revolve from an angle instead of a side.

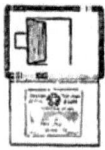

Similar experiments may be made with other figures, and the entire lesson devoted to observation of the facts which illustrate the following rule:

Rule 1. Any plane or line which is not at right angles to a line from its centre to the eye, is foreshortened, and does not appear its true dimensions.

NOTE 1. — A surface is at right angles to the direction in which it is seen when its opposite corners are equally distant from the eye. A line is at right angles to the direction in which it is seen when its ends are equally distant from the eye.

NOTE 2. — If any pupils are unable to trace the appearance of the square while holding the slate on the level of the eye, they may observe the appearance, and then place the slate in the usual position and draw from memory. This drawing may then be tested by placing the square at the back of the slate, and holding both in their original positions.

Lesson II. — Parallel and Equal Lines not Foreshortened, and Vertical Lines.

Draw the square B upon the slate, as explained in Lesson I. Its vertical edges appear unequal, and illustrate Rule 2.

Rule 2. The nearer of two parallel and equal lines which are not foreshortened appears the longer.

Place the drawing in the book to illustrate the rule. Drawings may be traced from the slate to thin paper, and then transferred to the book by tracing or any other means.

Unless directions to the contrary are given, all tracings made during these lessons are to be transferred to the drawing-book to illustrate the rules printed therein.

Trace the vertical lines of a cube or prism placed on the desk and near the eye, to illustrate the following rule. (This tracing may be omitted in the book.)

Rule 3. Vertical lines appear to converge when they are above or below the level of the eye, but their convergence is not represented, and vertical edges are always represented by vertical lines.

Lesson III. — The Horizontal Circle.

Hold the circular tablet horizontally and at the level of the eye. Then draw its appearance upon the slate.

Place the tablet horizontally upon a block or upon books at the back of the desk, and trace its appearance upon the slate. The slate should rest upon the desk and be held at the proper angle by the left hand.

Place the tablet upon the desk, and trace its appearance.

The distance between the eye and the object and between the eye and the slate should be the same for both tracings.

The tracings illustrate the following rules:

Rule 4. The horizontal circle appears a horizontal straight line when it is at the level of the eye. When below or above this level, the horizontal circle always appears an ellipse whose long axis is a horizontal line.

Rule 5. The farther above or below the level of the eye a horizontal circle is placed, the wider it appears. The short axis of the ellipse representing a horizontal circle changes its length as the circle is raised or lowered. The long axis is always represented of the same length, whatever the level of the circle.

NOTE. — The level of the circle remaining the same, its apparent width changes with the distance of the eye from the circle.

Lesson IV. — Parallel Lines.

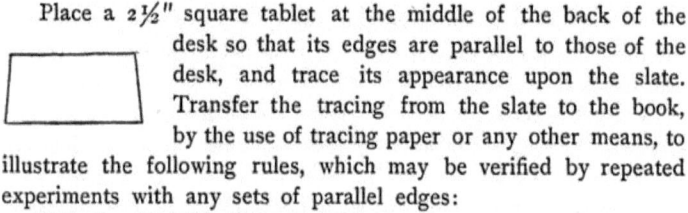

Place a 2½″ square tablet at the middle of the back of the desk so that its edges are parallel to those of the desk, and trace its appearance upon the slate. Transfer the tracing from the slate to the book, by the use of tracing paper or any other means, to illustrate the following rules, which may be verified by repeated experiments with any sets of parallel edges:

Rule 6. Parallel retreating edges appear to vanish, that is, converge toward a point.

NOTE. — Retreating edges are those which have one end nearer the eye than the other. Upon solids the farther end of any edge is a point of an invisible surface of the object.

Rule 7. Parallel edges which are parallel to the slate, that is, at right angles to the direction in which they are seen, do not appear to converge, and any parallel edges whose ends are at equal distances from the eye appear actually parallel.

Lesson V. — Parallel Retreating Horizontal Lines.

Place a large book horizontally at the middle of the back of the desk, with its edges parallel to those of the desk and its bound edge towards the pupil. Place a string under the upper cover of the book, and close against the binding. Hold 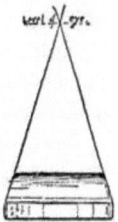 the left end of the string in the right hand, so that it appears to cover the left retreating edge of the book. At the same time, hold the right end of the string with the left hand, so that it appears to cover the right edge of the book. When both edges are covered, look at the point where the two parts of the string cross, and see that it is on the level of the eye. This illustrates the rule:

Rule 8. Parallel retreating horizontal edges appear to vanish at the level of the eye.

Trace upon the slate the lines of two walls as seen when looking 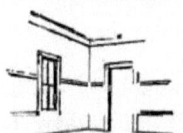 into a corner of the schoolroom. Trace the lines at the ceiling and those at the top and bottom of the blackboard. This tracing and that of the square and book below the eye illustrate the following rule :

Rule 9. Horizontal retreating lines above the eye appear to descend or vanish downward, and horizontal retreating lines below the eye appear to ascend or vanish upward. The vanishing point of any set of parallel retreating horizontal lines is at the level of the eye.

Lesson VI. — The Square.

Place a square tablet at the middle of the back of the desk, with its edges parallel to those of the desk. Two of the edges are not foreshortened, and are represented by parallel horizontal lines. The other edges vanish at a point over the tablet, and on the level of the eye.

Now place the tablet so that its edges are not parallel to those of the desk, and trace its appearance on the slate. None of the edges appear horizontal, and when the lines of the trac- 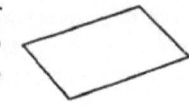 ing are continued as far as the slate will allow, the fact that they converge will be readily seen, and the drawing illustrates the following rule:

Rule 10. When one line of a right angle vanishes toward the right, the other line vanishes toward the left.

The drawing also shows that the edges appear of unequal length, and make unequal angles with a horizontal line, and illustrates the following rule :

Rule 11. When two sides of a square retreat at unequal angles, the one which is more nearly parallel to the picture plane (the slate) appears the longer, and more nearly horizontal.

Now turn the square so that its edges are at equal angles with the edges of the desk, and trace its edges and its diagonals. The two

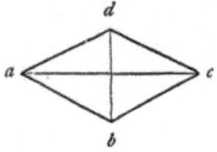

lower lines of the drawing *ab* and *bc* make equal angles with the edge of the slate, and also the two upper lines *cd* and *da*, but the angles of the upper lines are not the same as those of the lower lines. One diagonal of the square is represented by a vertical line, and

the other by a horizontal line. This drawing illustrates the following rules :

Rule 12. When the two lines of a horizontal right angle extend to right and left at equal angles with the picture plane, they are represented by lines which make equal angles with a horizontal line.

Rule 13. When the sides of a horizontal square are at equal angles with the picture plane, the nearer ones appear of equal length, and at equal angles with a horizontal line, and the same is true of the farther sides. One diagonal of the square appears a horizontal line, and the other appears a vertical line.

Conversely: When one diagonal of a horizontal square appears vertical, the other appears horizontal, and the nearer and farther sides appear at respectively equal angles with a horizontal line.

Lesson VII. — The Appearance of Equal Spaces on Any Line.

Cut from paper a square of three inches, and draw its diagonals. Place this square horizontally at the middle of the back of the desk, with its edges parallel to those of the desk, and then trace its appearance and its diagonals upon the slate.

Note. — The diagonals of a square bisect each other and give the centre of the square.

Compare the distance from the nearer end (1) of either diagonal to the centre of the square (2) with that from the centre of the square to the farther end of the diagonal (3), for an illustration of the following rule :

Rule 14. Equal distances on any retreating line appear unequal, the nearer of any two appearing the longer.

Transfer the tracing from the slate to the book.

Lesson VIII. — The Triangle.

Draw upon an equilateral triangular tablet a line from an angle to the centre of the opposite side. (This line is called an altitude.)

Connect the triangular tablet with the square tablet, and place them on the desk so that the base of the triangle is foreshortened, and its altitude is vertical. Trace the triangle and its altitude upon the slate. The tracing illustrates the fact that the nearer half of a receding line appears longer than the farther half (see Rule 14), and also the following rule :

Rule 15. The upper angle of a vertical isosceles or equilateral triangle, whose base is horizontal, appears in a vertical line erected at the perspective centre of the base.

Lesson IX. — The Prism.

Connect two square tablets by a rod to represent a cube, and hold the object so that one tablet only is visible, and discover that it must appear its real shape, *A*. This illustrates the following rule :

Rule 16. When one face only of a prism is visible, it appears its real shape.

Place the cube represented by tablets in the middle of the back of the desk, and trace its appearance. First, when two faces only of the solid would be visible, *B*, and second, when three faces would be seen, *C*. These tracings illustrate the following rule :

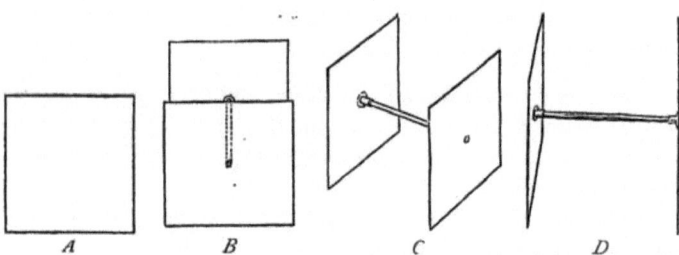

Rule 17. When two or more faces of a cube are seen, none of them can appear their real shapes.

Place the cubical form on the desk, with the tablets vertical, and one of them seen edgewise, *D*, and discover that the other tablet does not appear a straight line.   This illustrates the following rule :

Rule 18.   Only one end of a prism can appear a straight line at any one time.

Lesson X. — The Cylinder.

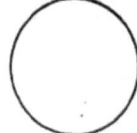

Connect two circular tablets by a 2½ " stick, to represent the cylinder. Hold the object so that one end only is visible, and see that it appears a circle. (See Rule 16.)

Place the object on the desk, so that its axis is horizontal but appears a vertical line, and trace its appearance.   The tracing illustrates the following rule :

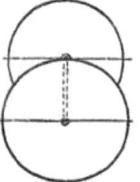

Rule 19.   When an end and the curved surface of a cylinder are seen at the same time, the end must appear an ellipse.

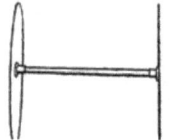

Place the object horizontally, and so that one end appears a vertical line, and trace to illustrate the following rule :

Rule 20.   When one end of a cylinder appears a straight line, the other appears an ellipse.

Place the object upright on the desk, and trace its ends and axis. Draw the long diameters of the ellipses, and discover that they are at right angles to the axis of the cylinder. This illustrates the following rules :

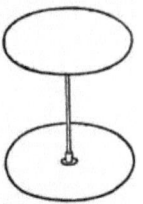

Rule 21. The bases of a vertical cylinder appear horizontal ellipses. The nearer base always appears the narrower ellipse.

Place the object with its axis horizontal and at an angle, so that

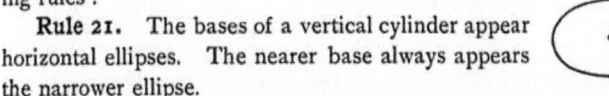

the surfaces of both tablets are visible. Trace the tablets and the rod, and then draw the long diameters of the ellipses, and discover that they are at right angles to the axis of the cylindrical form. The axes of the ellipses are inclined, and the drawing illustrates the following rules:

Rule 22. The bases of a cylinder appear ellipses whose long diameters are at right angles to the axis of the cylinder, the nearer base appearing the narrower ellipse.

NOTE.— The farther end may appear narrower than the nearer, but must always appear proportionally a wider ellipse than the nearer end.

Rule 23. Vertical foreshortened circles below or above the level of the eye appear ellipses whose axes are not vertical lines.

Rule 24. The long axis of an ellipse representing a vertical circle below or above the level of the eye is at right angles to the axis of a cylinder of which the circle is an end.

Rule 25. The elements of the cylinder appear to converge in the direction of the invisible end. This convergence is not represented when the cylinder is vertical.

NOTE 1.— Less than half the curved surface of the cylinder is visible at any one time.

NOTE 2.— The elements of the cylinder appear tangent to the bases and must always be represented by straight lines tangent to the ellipses which represent the bases. When the elements converge, the tangent points are not in the long axes of the ellipses. See illustration opposite Rule 19, in which if a straight line tangent to the ellipses be drawn, the tangent points will be found above the long axes of the ellipses.

Lesson XI. — The Cone.

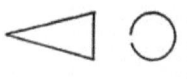

Hold the cone so that its axis is directed towards the eye and the cone appears a circle. Hold the cone so that its base appears a straight line, and it appears a triangle.

Place a circular tablet having a rod attached, to represent the axis of the cone, so that the axis is first vertical, and second inclined. Trace both positions of the object, and discover that the appearance of the circle is the same as in the case of the cylinder. The tracings illustrate the rule.

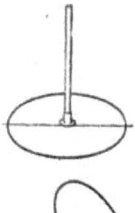

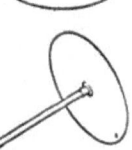

Rule 26. When the base of the cone appears an ellipse, the long axis of the ellipse is perpendicular to the axis of the cone.

NOTE 1. — More than half the curved surface of the cone will be seen when the vertex is nearer the eye than the base, and less than half will be seen when the base is nearer the eye than the vertex. The visible curved surface of the cone may range from all to none. See illustrations on p. 77.

NOTE 2. — The contour elements of the cone are represented by straight lines tangent to the ellipse which represents the base, and the points of tangency are not in the long axis of this ellipse. See illustrations on p. 77.

Lesson XII. — The Regular Hexagon.

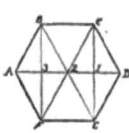

In this figure the opposite sides are parallel and equal. The long diagonal *A D* is parallel to the sides *B C* and *E F*, and it is divided into four equal parts by the short diagonals *B F* and *C E*, and by the long diagonal *B E* or *C F*.

The perspective drawing of this figure will be corrected by giving the proper vanishing to the different sets of parallel lines, and by making the divisions on the diagonal *A D* perspectively equal.

Draw the long and short diagonals upon a large hexagonal tablet. Place this tablet in a horizontal or vertical position, and then trace upon the slate its appearance and the lines upon it. The tracing illustrates the following rule :

Rule 27. In a correct drawing of the regular hexagon, any long diagonal, when intersected by a long diagonal and two short diagonals, will be divided into four equal parts.

Lesson XIII. — The Centre of the Ellipse does not Represent the Centre of the Circle. (*For teachers only.*)

Cut from paper a square of three inches, after having inscribed a circle in the square. Draw the diameters of the square and then place the square horizontally at the middle of the back of the desk, with its edges parallel to those of the desk. Trace the square, its diameters, and the inscribed circle, upon the slate. The circle appears an ellipse, and as the long axis of an ellipse bisects the short, it is evident that it must come below the centre of the square, and we discover that the centre of the ellipse does not represent the centre of the circle, and that the diameter of the circle appears shorter than a chord of the circle.

Lesson XIV. — Concentric Circles.

Cut a 4″ square from practice paper, and draw the diagonals. With the centre of the square as centre, draw two concentric circles, 4″ and 2″ in diameter.

Place the card horizontally upon the desk, as illustrated, and trace its appearance upon the slate, together with all the lines drawn upon it.

Draw the vertical line which is the short axis of both ellipses. Bisect the short axis of the outer ellipse, and draw the long axis *A* of this ellipse. Bisect the short axis of the inner ellipse, and draw its long axis *B*. It will be seen that the long axes are parallel, but do not coincide, and that both are in front of the point which represents the centre of the circles.

Each diameter of the larger circle is divided into four equal parts. The four equal spaces on the diameter which appears the short axis appear unequal according to Rule 14. The diameter which is parallel to the long axes of the ellipses has four equal spaces upon it, and they appear equal. This diameter is behind the long axes, but generally a very short distance, and in practice, if the distance *1, 2* between the ellipses measured on the long axis is one-fourth of the entire long axis, then the distance between the ellipses measured on the short axis must be a perspective fourth of the entire short axis. This illustrates the rule:

Rule 28. Foreshortened concentric circles appear ellipses whose short axes coincide. The distance between the ellipses on the short axis is perspectively the same proportion of the entire short axis, as the distance between the ellipses measured on the long axis, is geometrically of the entire long axis.

Lesson XV. — Vase Forms.

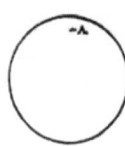

Place a sphere on the desk below the eye, and having marked the highest point upon it *A*, see that this point does not appear in the circle which defines the sphere, but comes below or inside this circle, a distance which varies with the distance of the sphere from and below the eye.

Place the modeled sphere, from which a small section has been cut, so that the section is horizontal and at the top, and trace the appearance of the object upon the slate. Indicate the elements of a cylinder or cone tangent to the ellipse which represents the section.

The circular section appears an ellipse, and appears inside the circle which defines the sphere. This illustrates the following rule:

Rule 29. In vase forms, when a cylindrical or conical body intersects a larger curved body or portion of convex form, and the line of intersection is visible in any position of the object, the contour lines of the smaller part extend inside the contour of the larger part: thus the extremities of the long axis of the ellipse which represents the intersection are not in the contour of the larger part.

Lesson XVI.—Frames.

In the frames are found regular concentric polygons with parallel sides, the angles of the inner polygons being in straight lines connecting the angles of the outer polygon with its centre. In polygons having an even number of sides, the lines containing the angles of the polygons form diagonals of the figures, as in the square.

In polygons having an odd number of sides, the lines containing the angles of the polygon are perpendicular to the sides opposite the angles, as in the triangle. The figures illustrate the above facts and the rule.

Draw upon large triangular and square tablets the lines shown in Figs. *A* and *B*. Place the tablets horizontally on the desk, or

 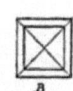   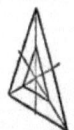 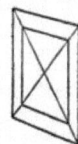

A.　　B.　　C.　　D.

support them vertically, and trace upon the slate the appearance of their edges and all the lines drawn upon them. The tracings illustrate Rule 30.

Rule 30. In representing the regular frames, the angles of the inner figure must be in straight lines passing from the angles of the outer figure to the centre. These lines are altitudes or diagonals of the polygons.

NOTE. — The most important principles of the subject are stated briefly and simply in this chapter for the benefit of teachers of elementary work. Teachers of art schools and advanced classes will find the subject treated at greater length, and in a way suited to the requirements of advanced students, in the book, "*Free-hand Drawing, Light and Shade, and Free-hand Perspective,*" by Anson K. Cross.

DRAWINGS ILLUSTRATING THE RULES.

The principles governing the appearance of geometric forms have been illustrated by the use of tablets. The following drawings represent both tablets and solid objects in different positions, which illustrate the rules.

The first drawings represent tablets and objects when placed upon the pupils' desks. When objects are thus placed perspective effects are often unpleasant ; therefore after the first experiments the objects should be raised from the desk. They should not be placed so as to be foreshortened less than the first objects represented below.

The drawings are reproductions of pen sketches. Some are slightly accented, but they are not given for examples of handling, for which the sketches of the pupils' drawing books must be used.

The figures in which light lines are found illustrate the appearance which drawings should have before any lines have been erased.

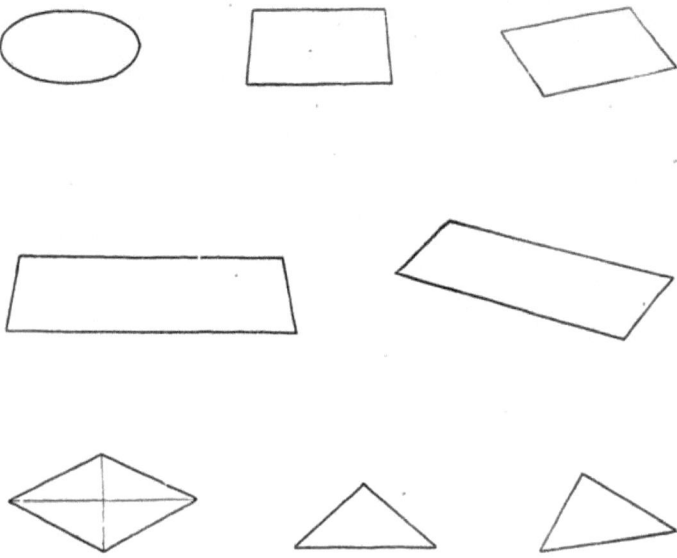

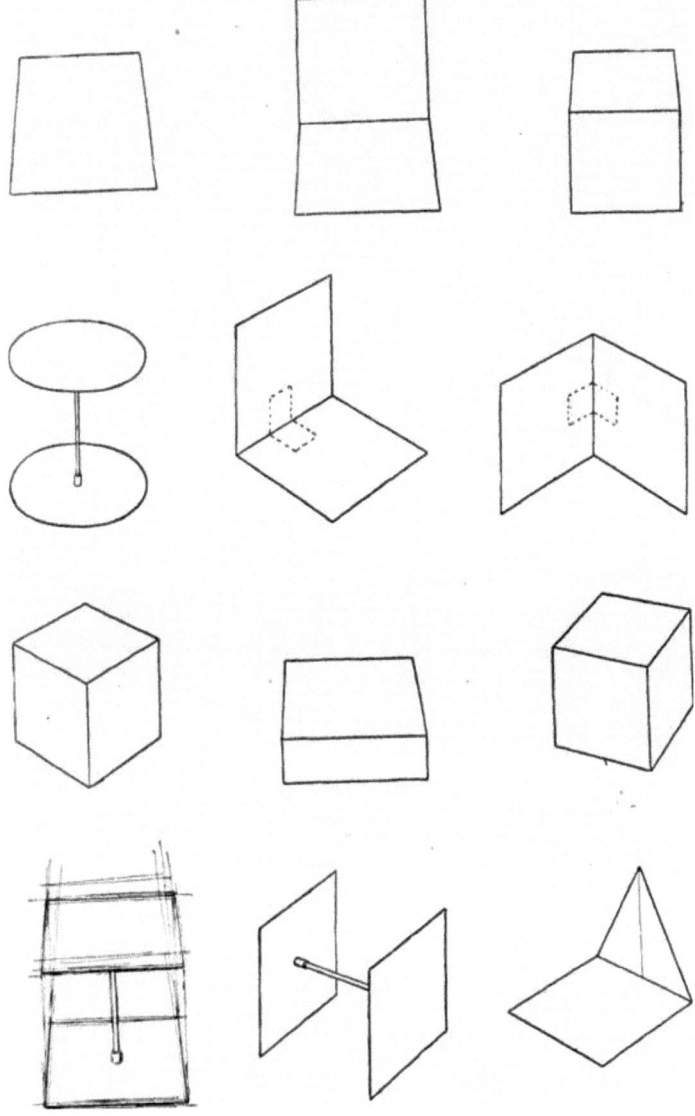

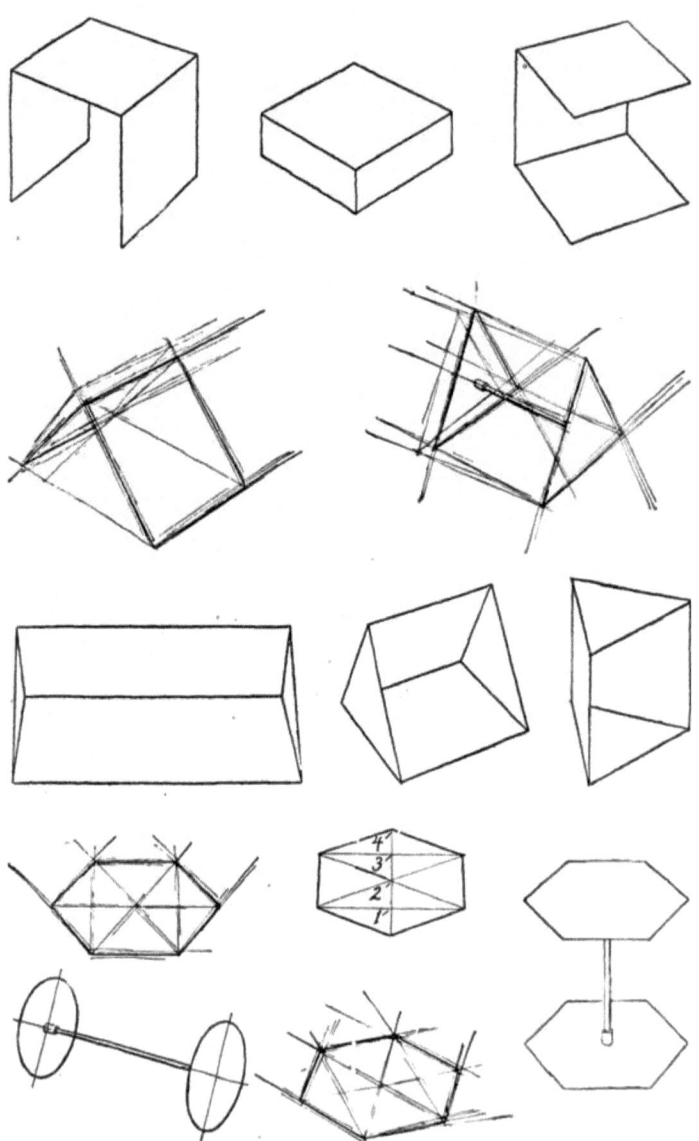

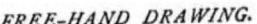

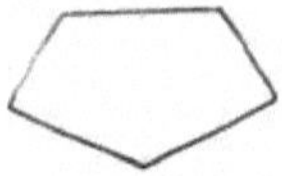

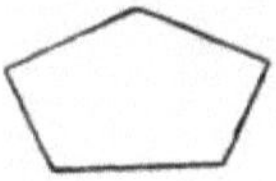

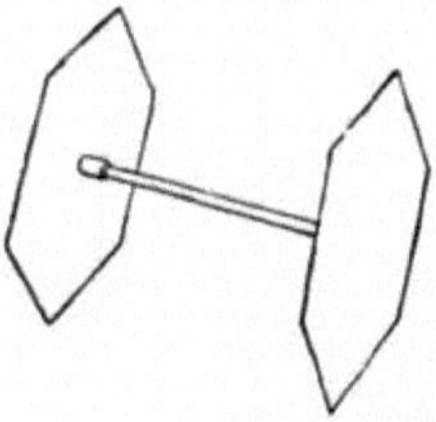

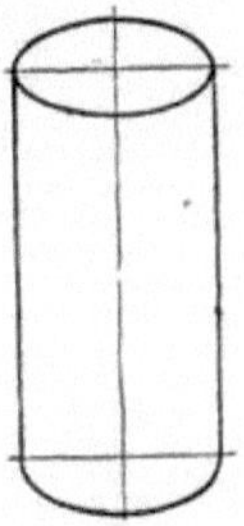

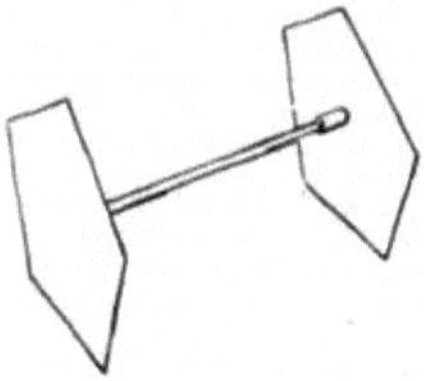

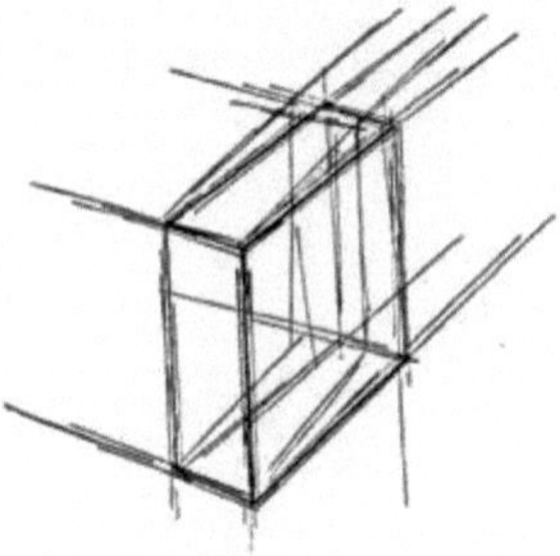

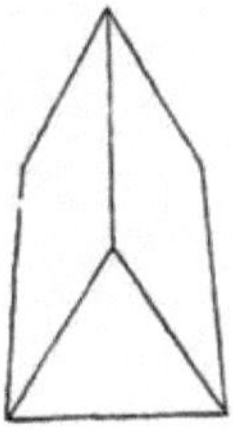

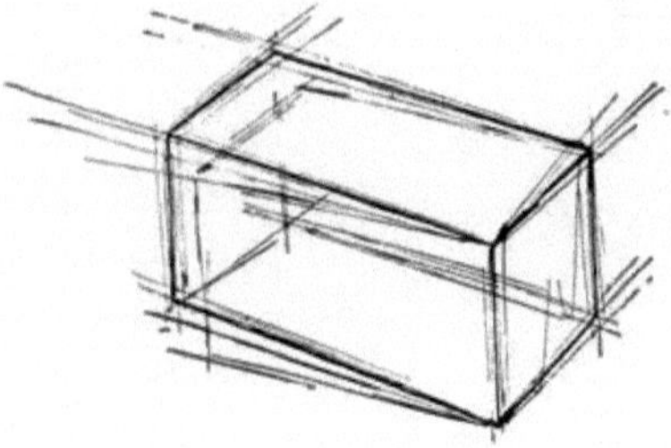

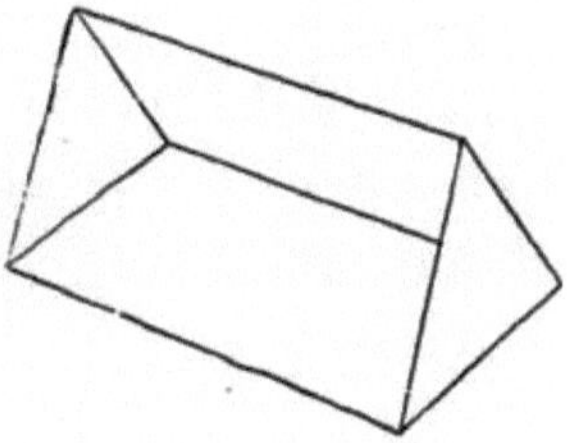

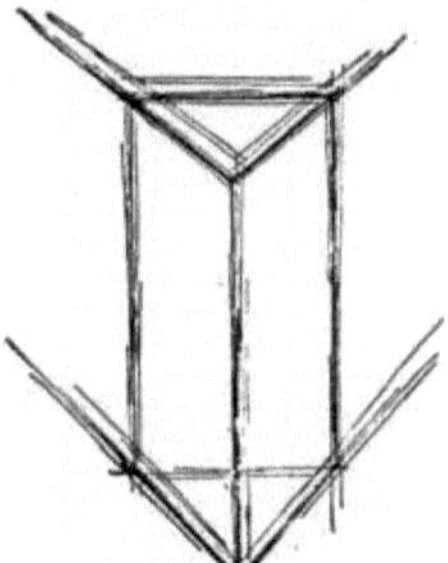

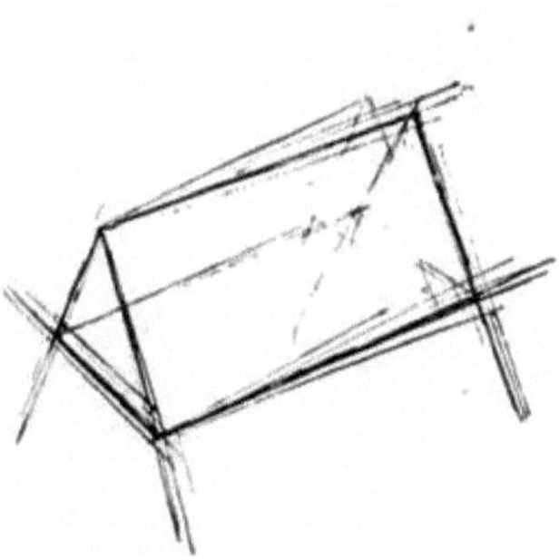

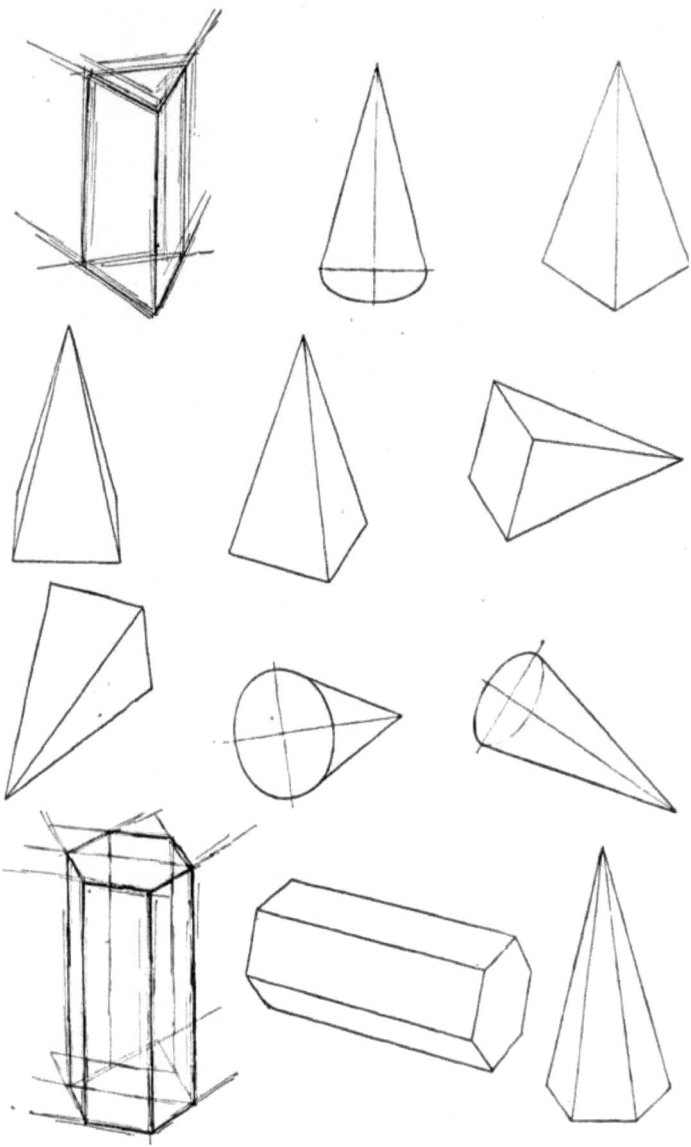

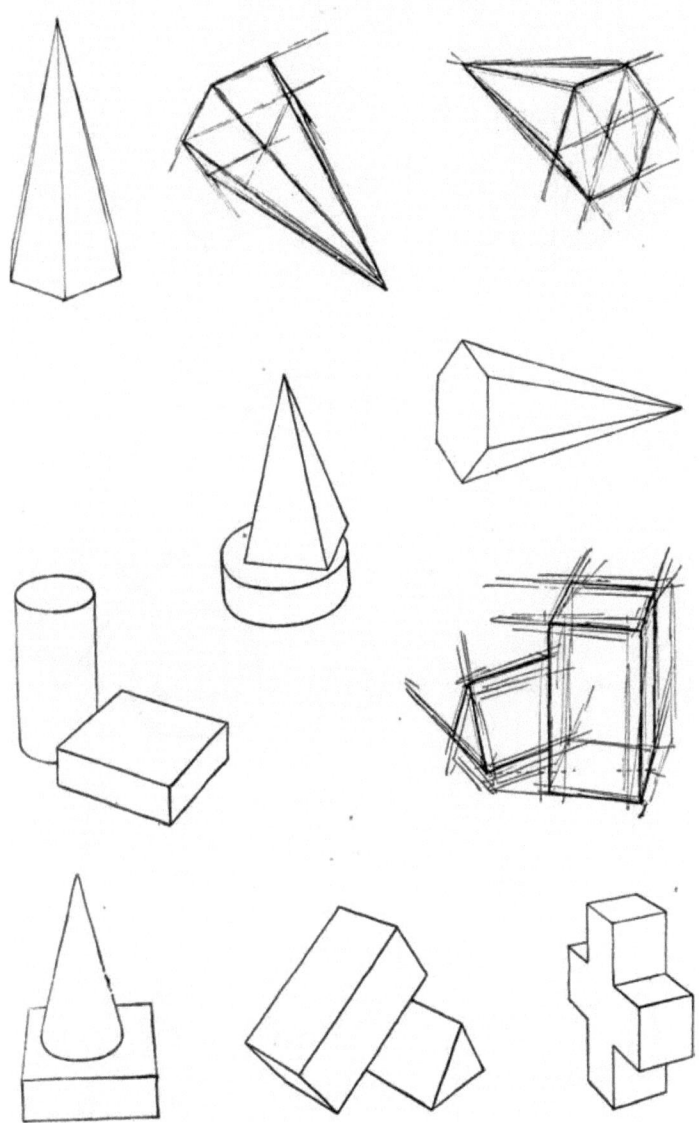

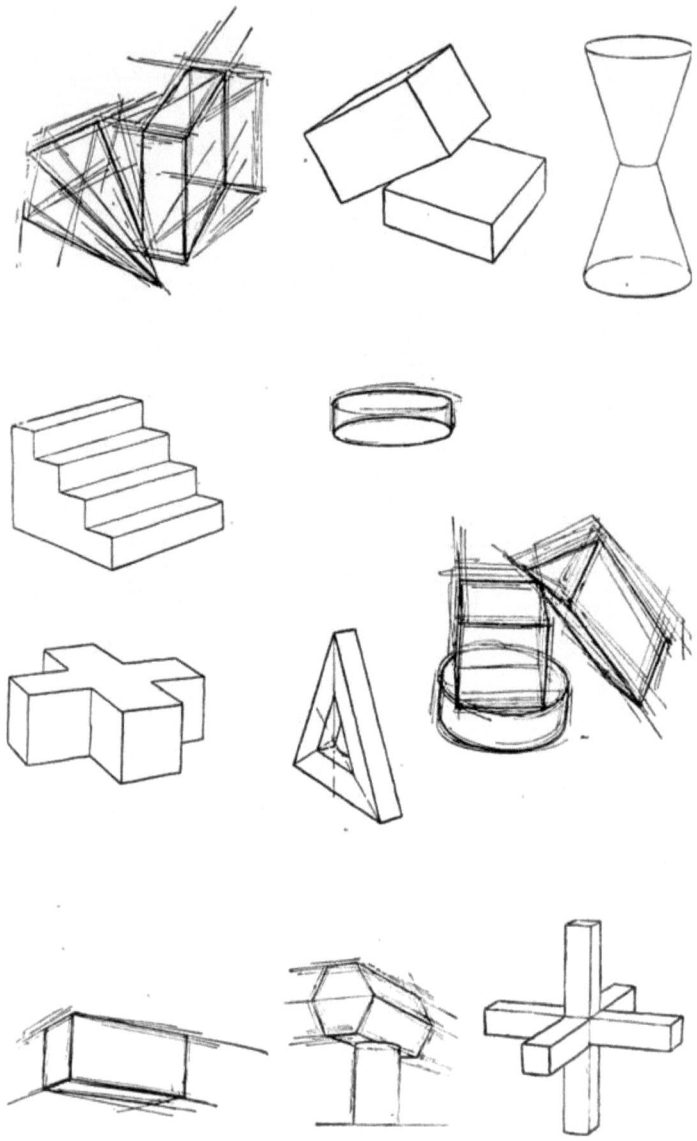

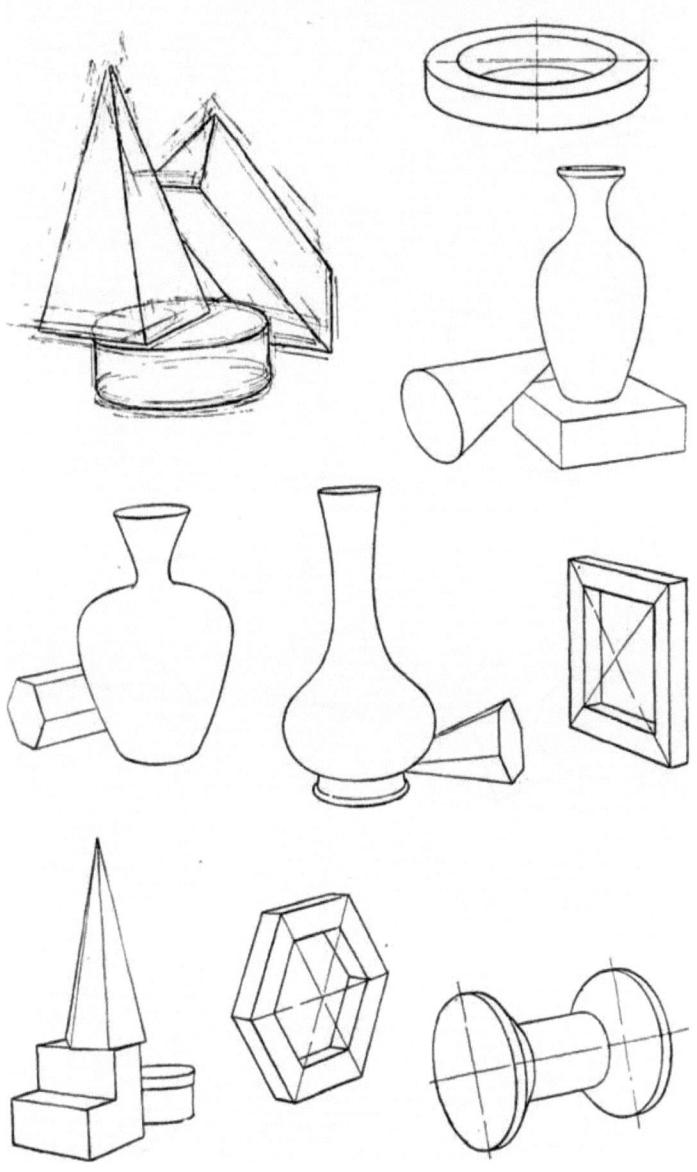

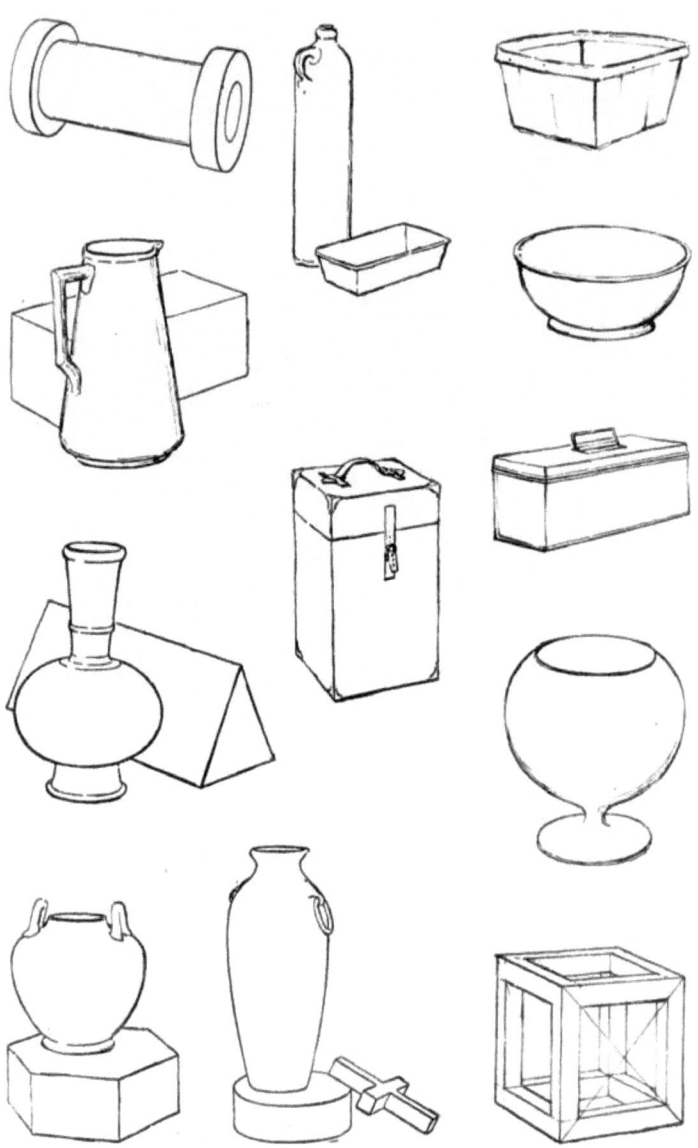

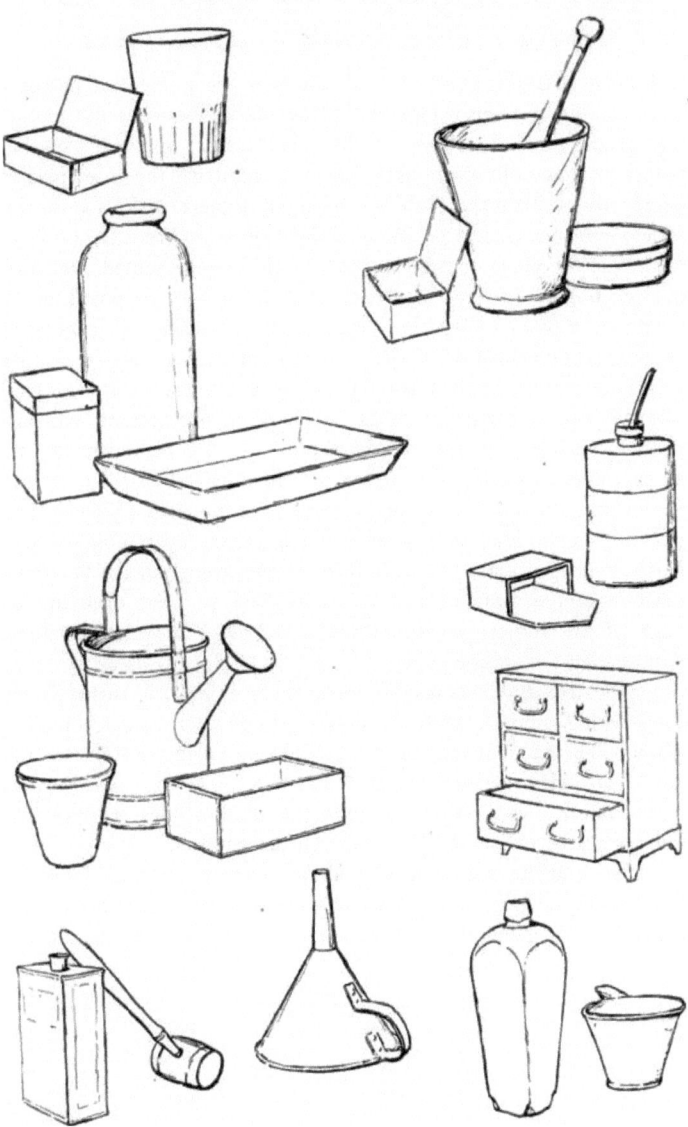

CHAPTER VII.

SCIENTIFIC PERSPECTIVE AND MODEL DRAWING.

(This chapter is for teachers of drawing and advanced art students.)

A PERSPECTIVE is generally understood to be a scientific perspective made upon a vertical picture plane placed between the eye of the spectator and the subject to be represented. Drawings of this nature are generally made upon paper by applying the principles of perspective. To make such a drawing it is necessary to know the forms, dimensions, and positions of the objects, to know the position of the picture plane on which they are to be represented, and also the position of the eye of the spectator, which is supposed to be fixed at one point called the *station-point*. Scientific perspective is as exact as geometry,— in fact it is a branch of geometry, and its principles may be applied upon paper to a drawing of any subject, so exact that if the paper could be rendered transparent, and suspended vertically in the position of the picture plane, every line upon it would be found to appear to coincide with the line of the object which it represents when the eye is at the station-point. The drawing is, in fact, just what would be given by tracing upon a vertical sheet of glass placed in front of the group, and in the given position of the assumed picture plane, lines to cover each line or edge of the subject as seen through the glass and from the fixed point called the station-point.

Perspective drawings may be made upon cylindrical surfaces, but the drawing generally made is supposed to be upon a vertical picture plane. The student may readily produce a drawing to illustrate the nature of a plane perspective by fixing the eye at one point in front of a window, and then tracing upon the window lines to cover the lines of whatever may be seen through the window.

Artists and illustrators have made perspective drawings for many hundred years; and these drawings have quite generally been satisfactory when geometric forms have been represented ; but in the highest art, which represents the human figure, artists have not made scientific perspective drawings, but have drawn instead by eye the actual appearance of each figure in the subject, and thus their drawings do not require to be seen from one fixed point in order that they may represent the appearance of all the figures.

In order to understand the difference between a scientific perspective and the drawing which an artist makes of a figure or other subject not architectural, we must determine first what the eye sees, and second any points of difference that may exist between what the eye sees and a plane perspective drawing.

The eye contains a lens whose action is the same as that of the lens found in a camera. The rays of light from any object to the

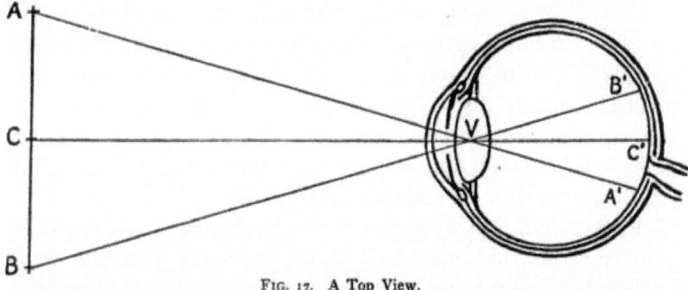

FIG. 17. A Top View.

eye pass through its lens and are focussed by it upon the sensitive nerves at the back of the eye. The surface of the eye which receives the light transmitted by the lens is spherical, and the rays of light pass through the lens and strike upon the sensitive retina in a direction practically perpendicular to the surface of the retina (Fig. 17).

Most of the inner surface of the eye is sensitive to the rays of light, and so the eye sees a very wide field of view. If the eye is fixed upon any object directly in front of the spectator, objects above, below, to the left, and to the right will be seen at one time, but all very indistinctly ; and though the spectator may be conscious of seeing objects at almost the extreme right and left of his position, they will be seen so indistinctly that they will not be recognized. A very small space is seen distinctly at any one time. Thus, in reading this book, it will be impossible to read a word at the left of any line and distinguish a letter at the right of the line, and only a few letters can be read without motion of the eye. The field of distinct vision is thus confined to a very small visual angle. By this is meant that the rays which come from the extreme points of what is clearly seen form very small angles with each other, and the eye cannot bring to a focus upon the retina all the rays from any object which causes large visual angles.

The rays coming to the eye from any object form a conical body whose vertex is in the lens of the eye ; passing through the lens the rays form a conical body whose vertex is also in the lens. The central visual ray, or the axis of both the cones, is perpendicular to the surface of the retina which receives it ; and the whole cone of rays which gives the image of the object is intersected by the curved surface of the retina practically at right angles to all the rays. The proportions which any object appears to have are thus dependent upon the angles between the visual rays, and the arc which measures the angle between any two rays, as those from A and B, Fig. 17, will nearly coincide with the surface of the retina.

All objects are seen by means of the images which they produce upon the retina; but any one is clearly seen only when the eye is directed to it, and thus we must accept this distinct image formed in the eye as the true picture, — that is, as the true appearance of the object.

The retina has the general shape of a sphere, but the part that receives the rays which form a sharp image is so small that its curvature is very slight, and the image upon it is practically the same as that which would be given upon a plane surface at right angles to the axis of the cone of visual rays ; and we see that for all practical purposes we may speak of a true picture, meaning one which is similar in its form to the image of the eye, as produced by intersecting the cone of visual rays by a plane perpendicular to the central ray.

By appearance we mean, then, the image which any object produces upon the retina, and a picture which represents this appearance is a true picture. By represents is meant a picture which is similar, geometrically, to the image, so that the picture will cause in the eye the same image that the object would produce if the object were seen instead of its true picture.

The limit to the visual angle within which clear vision is possible is very small, and to see almost any object clearly the eye moves so as to be directed to its different parts ; but any object which does not create visual angles greater than 30° will be so pictured upon the retina that when its central part is clearly seen the image is but slightly different from that which is given by intersecting the cone of visual rays by a plane perpendicular to the central visual ray instead of by the curved surface of the eye.

We must generally draw upon paper or some other flat surface, and the problem for the artist is to produce upon a plane a drawing which shall cause in the eye the nearest possible approach to the image on the curved surface of the eye which is produced by the object itself.

Seeing is a matter of education principally, and it is immaterial what the image in the eye actually is in regard to the relations of its details, for the mind reads the images by referring to the facts remembered concerning previous and similar images. Authorities on perspective state that straight lines appear curved, — that is, cause curved images in the eye ; but it is of no consequence to the artist whether the images are curved or not, for admitting that the images are curved, the eyes of all read the images as those of straight lines, the mind supplying the knowledge of straightness whenever the images are produced by lines which are known to be straight. When curved images in the eye are produced by lines which are not known to be straight, the mind receives the impression of curved lines in nature, and the artist would represent the lines by curved lines ; but if he represents by curved lines lines which the mind knows to be straight, his drawing will not create the same impression as the image in the eye caused by the actual lines ; for if the images of the eye are curved the mind does not know it and reads them always as straight. The eye is simply a mechanical instrument, and we see much more through the mind than by study of the proportions of the image in the eye as if it were a drawing or a map.

The problem for the artist is, then, to produce a drawing which shall, as nearly as possible, cause in the eye the same visual angles as the object, and which shall at the same time cause the mind to bring forward, as far as possible, the same ideas concerning the object that the object represented would create; and this drawing must be made upon a plane surface.

Having decided that the image in the eye — the appearance of the object — must be considered a true picture of the object, and that it is practically what is given by intersecting the visual rays by a plane perpendicular to them, — that is, to the central ray to any object, we will study the drawings which are given upon the vertical picture plane, generally used in scientific perspective, to discover any points of difference between them and what the eye sees. The illustrations used will generally be from photographs, for the camera gives an exact perspective drawing in which the negative corresponds to the picture plane and the centre of the lens to the station-point.

All the illustrations of this chapter, except those in outline, are reproduced directly from photographs. Photographs which represent objects causing visual angles greater than 30° are always distortions, and when the visual angles represented are as large as 60° or 90° the distortions are generally very noticeable and very unpleasant. Photographs taken with lenses which include angles of from 60° to 90° are as common as those which represent smaller angles and thus give more nearly what the eye sees. The photographs from which the illustrations of this chapter are taken do not distort more than the photographs and illustrations which are always to be found in the common representations of interiors and exteriors, and often such representations present greater distortions than these illustrations.

The illustrations of this chapter are smaller than the original photographs, and thus they should be seen from a shorter distance than the photographs. But still they are not more distorted than many drawings which are made for illustrations by those who make scientific perspective drawings instead of drawing by eye, and by those who draw from nature with the false ideas of the appearance of form which are given by study of scientific perspective without that of the free-hand perspective; and often illustrative drawings are more distorted than those of this chapter.

Fig. 18 is from a photograph of a sphere which was placed directly below the camera and upon a horizontal surface. The camera was horizontal, so the negative — that is, the picture plane — was

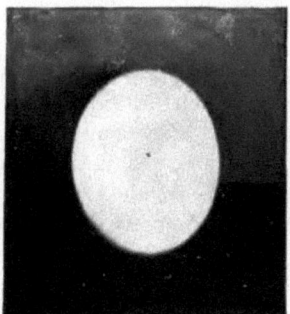

FIG. 18. Perspective of a Sphere. From Photograph.

vertical. The picture of the sphere is seen to be a vertical ellipse, and it does not create a satisfactory impression of the round object.

Fig. 19 is a side view representing the sphere, the eye, and a vertical picture plane touching the sphere. The visual rays from the sphere to the eye form a cone, and Fig. 19 shows that this cone of rays is intersected obliquely by the vertical picture plane. The cone is a circular cone, — that is, if it is cut by a plane at right angles to its axis the sections will be a circle; and by geometry we know that if it is cut by a plane not at right angles to the axis, as is the picture plane in the figure, the section will be an ellipse. This elliptical section is the picture of the sphere on the vertical picture plane, and the ellipse covers the sphere when the eye is at the station-point, — that is, the ellipse appears a circle whose image coincides with the circular image produced in the eye by the sphere. When the eye is in the proper position for viewing Fig. 18, it appears a circle, and if the eye is

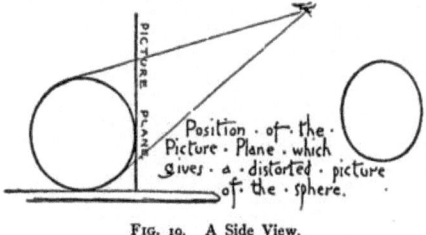

FIG. 19.   A Side View.

placed at a point about 4¼″ from the paper and in a perpendicular to the page erected at the point marked *CV*, the ellipse of Fig. 18 will be seen obliquely and foreshortened into a circle.[1] In order to see the figure when the eye is so near, it will be necessary to make a circular hole about ⅛″ in diameter in a card and view the drawing through this hole, which serves as the station-point.

This illustrates the important fact that to create the same image in the eye that the object does, any perspective drawing must be seen from one fixed point, and if seen from any other point the perspective drawing will appear distorted, and create in the eye a very different image from that which the object itself will form.

Fig. 20 represents a sphere and a cube placed upon a horizontal surface below and at the left of the eye, — the camera. This picture does not cause the reader to think of a sphere, but it does create the idea of a cube, because cubes have been represented in this way so generally that the average person accepts the drawing as a satisfactory representation of the cube. But it is evident that if the inclined ellipse which represents the sphere, is a distortion, the representation of the cube below it must be as much distorted, and actually it is more distorted than the ellipse. If the eye is placed

---

[1] These letters are often used to designate the centre of vision, or the point on the picture exactly opposite the eye of the spectator. At this point all lines perpendicular to the picture plane vanish.

at the station-point, which for Fig. 20 is about 5⅛" from the paper and in a perpendicular to the page erected at the point marked *CV*, the drawing will be seen obliquely and so foreshortened that the

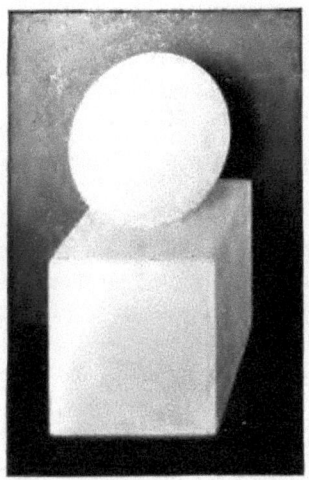

FIG. 20. Perspective of a Sphere and Cube.

ellipse will appear a circle, and the representation of the cube will cause the same image in the eye that the cube does. Figs. 18 and 20 are distorted because they are made on a vertical picture plane through which the visual rays pass obliquely.

Fig. 21 is a side view representing the sphere situated as in Fig. 18 with a picture plane touching the sphere, and so inclined

as to be perpendicular to a line from the spectator's eye to the centre
of the sphere. This line is the central visual ray and the axis of the
circular cone formed by the visual rays. Since this cone is intersected by a picture plane which is perpendicular to its axis, the
section of the cone — that is, the perspective or picture of the
sphere — is a true picture of the object and is similar in its form to
the picture formed by the sphere in the eye.

The picture of Fig. 21 is a circle, and differs from that of Fig. 18
in a very important point ; for when Fig. 18 is correctly seen the eye

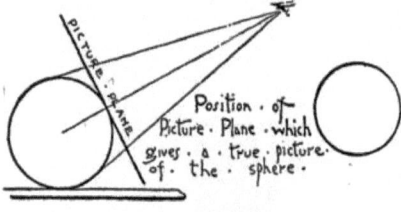

must be at one fixed point.
When thus seen it creates
in the eye a circular image,
but the picture of Fig. 21
may be seen from any
point situated in a perpendicular to the picture
erected at its centre, and
the image produced in the

FIG. 21. A Side View.

eye will be a circle, without regard to the distance of the eye from
the paper.

We must decide that the drawing, Fig. 21, which represents the
sphere by a circle is preferable to the drawing, Fig. 18, which
represents the sphere by an ellipse ; for though Fig. 18 may be seen
so as to create a circular image in the eye, there is little chance of
this occurring, and practically, no person, whether artist or not,
would ever think of drawing anything but a circle to represent a
sphere.

Perspective drawings are distorted as shown because any person
who looks at a drawing or picture naturally holds it in the hand, so
that its surface is at right angles to the direction in which it is seen ;
or, if it is a framed picture, the person stands directly in front of it,
and so that its surface is not foreshortened. If a picture is too large
to be taken in at a glance, the eye is moved so that when any part
is seen it is looked at from a direction practically perpendicular
to the surface. A person looking at a large canvas naturally places
himself in front of the left part when he is studying figures or other
details represented in this part ; and in the same way he studies

figures or detail at the extreme right of the canvas by standing directly in front of this part. Of course he obtains his impression of the effect of the whole picture when he is in front of the centre of the picture, but when in this position he does not study the extreme parts for detail because he has unconsciously acquired the habit of looking at a picture so that its surface is not foreshortened. Whether the eye moves or not in studying a large canvas is a question of no importance, for the artist never draws a figure distorted, as Figs. 18 and 20 are distorted, in order that it may look right when the picture is seen from one fixed point near the canvas; and he never makes a drawing which he intends to be seen obliquely from a point in a perpendicular to the picture which falls outside the limits of the drawing.

If the perspective drawings, Figs. 18, 19, and 20, are looked at naturally they will give very false ideas of the appearances of the objects they represent. In order that Fig. 18 give the impression of a circle, the page must be held vertically and so that the whole drawing is below the eye. If Fig. 20 is to give the right impression, the page must be held vertically and so that the whole drawing is below and at the left of the eye, and it is evident that, naturally, no person would ever make a free-hand drawing which must be viewed so unnaturally.

The cube shown in Fig. 20 is represented by a scientific perspective drawing in Fig. 22. This drawing will give the same image in the eye that the cube does if it is seen from a point about $9''$ from the paper erected at the point marked CV. The image produced in the eye by thus viewing Fig. 22 will be found to be practically the same as that given by looking at Fig. 23 from a perpendicular to the page erected at the centre of the drawing; and it is evident that the perspective, Fig. 22, when it is seen as it generally will be, is as much a distortion as the ellipse of Fig. 18 which represents the sphere.

To create the same image in the eye as the object, Fig. 20 must be seen from a point about $5\frac{1}{8}''$ from the paper, and this may cause the student to think the drawing more distorted than perspective drawings generally are. But this is not the case, for if the dimensions of the drawing are made twice as great, the distance of the eye will be about 10¼", and if the drawing is made three times the size, the distance of the eye will be increased proportionately and will be a normal distance, while the drawing is as distorted as Fig. 20 because it must be seen obliquely.

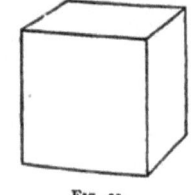

Fig. 22 is a scientific perspective which distorts much less than such drawings generally do, for the distance of the eye is greater in proportion to the size of the drawing than is often the case, so that there will generally be a greater difference between perspective drawings and model drawings than between Figs. 22 and 23.

FIG. 22.
Scientific Perspective.

Fig. 24 is a perspective drawing upon a vertical plane; it represents two horizontal circular plinths, *A* and *B*, *A* being directly in front and *B* placed at the right. This drawing represents the circles of the plinth at the left by horizontal ellipses. The eye sees these circles as horizontal ellipses, and the part *A* is a true picture, except that its height is too great.

FIG. 23.
Free-Hand Perspective.

The horizontal circles of plinth *B* are represented by inclined ellipses, and so, to give the right effect, the drawing must be seen from a point opposite *CV*, and about 4¾" from the paper. If seen naturally the part *B* does not form a true picture of the object, and horizontal circles should not be represented by inclined ellipses unless they are tangent to squares, or so placed that they cannot be represented as they appear, and give

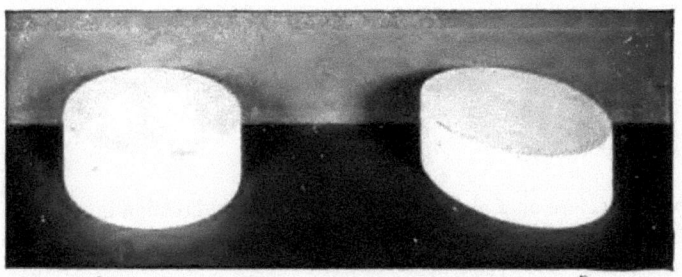

Fig. 24. Perspective of Circular Plinths.

the correct impression of their position. The plinths A and B are of the same size, but it will be noticed that the perspective of B is wider than that of A.

It appears that all depends upon the position of the station-point from which the drawing is to be seen, and that any drawing which requires to be foreshortened in order to look like the object is not a satisfactory representation. The artist naturally draws what will create a true picture in the eye when the drawing is seen perpendicularly, and any drawing of a single object which requires to be seen obliquely, cannot be accepted as the best picture of the object. The best picture of any object must be the one which, when not fore-shortened, causes in the eye an image practically like that which the object itself would produce.

Fig. 21 shows that the picture plane which gives a picture which is similar to the image in the eye must be at right angles to the direction in which the object is seen. In the case of the sphere below the eye, as in Fig. 21, a circle is given upon the inclined picture plane, and this circle, when viewed naturally, causes the same image in the eye that the sphere does; but it is possible to obtain

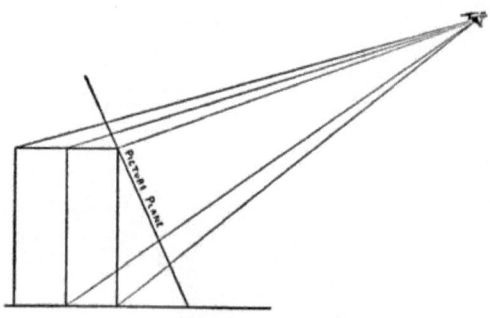

Fig. 26. A Side View.

a true picture on a plane at right angles to the direction in which an object is seen which will not when viewed naturally, produce a satisfactory impression of the object.

Fig. 25 is from a photograph of a vertical square prism below the eye, the picture plane (the negative) being at right angles to the direction in which the prism was seen as illustrated by the side view, Fig. 26. The side view shows that the lower ends of the vertical edges are farther from the eye than the upper ends; these vertical edges must then appear to converge downwards, just as Fig. 25 represents them. Fig. 25 is a plane perspective upon an inclined picture plane instead of a vertical plane. When the eye is at the station-point, which for Fig. 25 is about 4⅛" from the paper, and in a perpendicular to the page erected at the centre of the draw-ing, and when the drawing is inclined, as shown in Fig. 26, its lines will exactly cover the edges of the object, and will, of course, cause

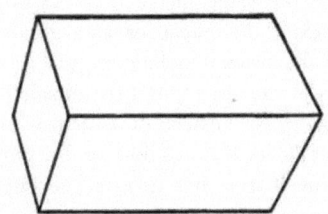

FIG. 28. Free-Hand Perspective.

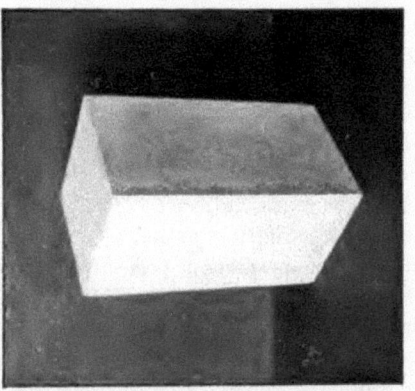

FIG. 25. Perspective on an Inclined Plane.

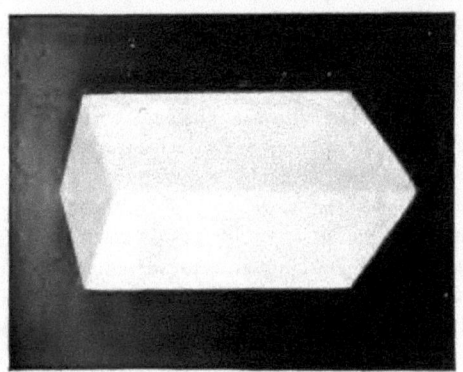

FIG. 27. Perspective on a Vertical Plane.

in the eye the same image that the object does; but if the eye is placed nearer the paper or at a greater distance, or if the paper is not at the proper inclination, the lines of Fig. 26 will not cover the edges of the object, and the drawing will give the impression of an inclined prism instead of a vertical one. This drawing is just as objectionable as Figs. 18 and 20, for it requires to be seen from one fixed point if it is not to give the impression of inclined lines in nature.

If the plane perspective drawing is made upon a vertical plane, the vertical edges will be represented by the vertical lines of Fig. 27; but to give the right impression of the relative height and width of the appearance, this drawing must be foreshortened by being seen from a point about $4\frac{1}{8}''$ from the paper and in a perpendicular to the page erected at *CV*. If looked at naturally the image created is too high, but it gives the right impression of the form and position of the object, and is more satisfactory than Fig. 25. We see that in the case of the prism, an exact perspective drawing on an inclined plane is not as satisfactory as one upon a vertical picture plane, for though giving the proportions correctly, it does not give the impression of a vertical object. Neither Fig. 25 nor Fig. 27 is satisfactory or would be made by the artist, who would represent the vertical edges by vertical lines, but would give the impression of the relative width and height by representing the visual proportions of the object. The artist works by feeling and by eye more than by measurement, but, in theory, the width to be represented by means of vertical lines would be the average of the widths at top and bottom of Fig. 25, — that is, the width would be measured at the centre of the object for comparison with the height, and the resulting drawing, Fig. 28, is like Fig. 27, but not so high.

The artist, as he draws any single object, does not think of a picture plane, but simply feels the visual proportions and represents the object so as to create a satisfactory impression of it and its position, and he represents vertical edges by vertical lines. Vertical edges appear to vanish just as much as do horizontal retreating edges, but they are not so represented for the reason explained. With this exception any single object causing small visual angles should be represented just as it appears, and its appearance is given upon a picture plane which is at right angles to the direction in which the object is seen. If the object is above the eye, the plane will incline at the top toward the eye; if the object is on the level of the eye, the plane will be vertical, and wherever the object is situated with reference to the spectator, whether in front, at the right, or at the left, the picture plane will be perpendicular to the direction in which the object is seen.

Generally, objects are so little above or below the level of the eye that a perspective, made upon a vertical plane at right angles to a horizontal line from the eye to a point just over or under the object, will be satisfactory, and if an object is far enough from the level of the eye to cause its perspective on this vertical plane to be much too high, the artist's drawing may be supposed to be made upon the vertical plane, and corrected by changing the height of the drawing to agree with the apparent height of the object. The question of the plane of the drawing is, however, of little importance when single objects are studied, for pupils should then always be taught to give the actual visual proportions, to represent vertical edges by vertical lines, and to take any measurements of proportions with the measuring rod always at right angles to the visual rays; and it is not necessary for them to think of picture planes, vertical or inclined.

All single objects causing small visual angles should generally be represented just as they appear except as to the convergence of vertical edges, but when there are several objects to be represented in the same drawing the problem is more complicated.

A row of three equal boxes placed in a straight line is represented by the Figs. 29, 30, and 31. Fig. 29 represents the actual appearance of the left box, Fig. 30 that of the central box, and Fig. 31 that of the right-hand box. Each drawing is a separate and complete picture, and should be studied when the other figures are covered by pieces of paper, and with the eye in a perpendicular to the drawing. When Fig. 29 is thus studied it gives the best impression of the appearance and position of the left box ; when Figs. 29 and 31 are covered, and Fig. 30 is seen perpendicularly, it gives the best representation of the central box ; and when Figs. 29 and 30 are covered, and Fig. 31 is seen perpendicularly, it gives the best impression of the box at the right. Box *A* is farther from the eye than

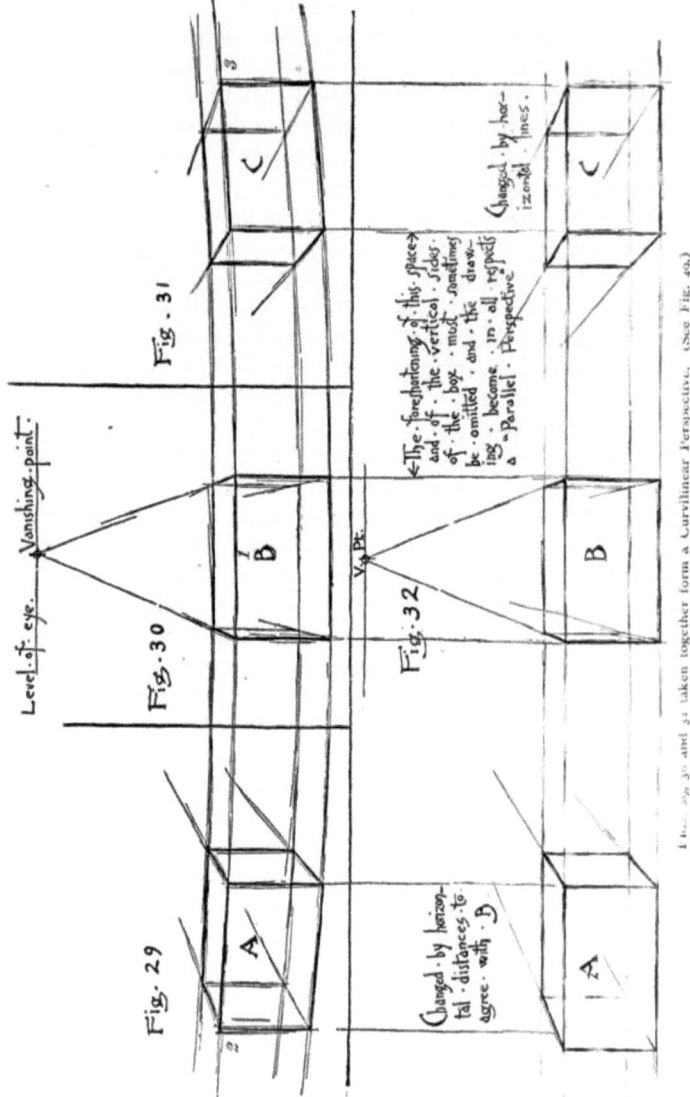

Level of eye.   Vanishing point.

Fig. 29

Fig. 30

Fig. 31

Fig. 32

V. Pt.

A   B   C

Changed by horizontal distances to agree with B

The foreshortening of this space and of the vertical sides of the box must sometimes be omitted and the drawing become in all respects a Parallel Perspective.

Changed by horizontal lines.

Figs. 29, 30 and 31 taken together form a Curvilinear Perspective. (See Fig. 40.)

box *B*, and, consequently, its vertical edges appear shorter than those of box *B*, and their ends appear respectively higher than those of the edges of box *B*. The ends of the long edges of the box *A* are unequally distant from the eye, and by Rule 6 they must appear to vanish; and by Rule 17 we find that not one of the three visible faces of the box *A* can appear its real shape. The same facts govern the appearance of box *C*, Fig. 31 ; and it is evident if we draw each of the boxes as it is seen, and with its corners relatively higher than the corresponding ones of box *B*, that we cannot look at the drawings, Figs. 29, 30, and 31, as one picture, for if the three are seen at one time, the impression of boxes arranged in a curved line is given.

These figures illustrate the fact that when objects, or an object, cause large visual angles (angles over 30°), we cannot draw the appearance of each object, or of each part of the one object, and produce a satisfactory picture, for the picture will give the appearance of the objects and not their relative positions. It is much more important that the one drawing, Fig. 32, which represents the three boxes, give the impression of boxes arranged in a straight line, than that the part representing the box at the left, or that at the right, be a true picture of the box; therefore, the artist who represents in one drawing the three boxes will do so by the use of horizontal straight lines, as in Fig. 32.

The boxes, *A* and *C* are farther from the eye than box *B*, consequently, their front faces are foreshortened horizontally, so as to appear narrower than that of *B*. In Fig. 32 the artist would generally represent the three faces of equal width, and he would, also, probably omit the representation of the foreshortening of the spaces between the boxes. The three front vertical faces are below the eye, and so foreshortened vertically; this foreshortening would not be represented in Fig. 32 unless the horizontal foreshortening is given, and generally, the artist would make for Fig. 32, an exact parallel perspective drawing, as illustrated and explained under Fig. 34.

Figs. 29, 30, and 31, when looked at incorrectly as one picture, give the effect of curved lines, and lead one to question if straight lines in nature do not appear curved. It is a fact that straight lines do appear curved, even when they are short. The line connecting the front upper edges of the three boxes, Figs. 29, 30, and 31, will prove this, if we apply Rules 6 and 9. Thus, point 1 is the nearer end of line 1–2, which must, by Rule 6, appear to incline upward to the left; and point 1 is the nearer end of line 1–3, which must then appear to incline upward to the right. But the line 2–1–3 appears horizontal at 1; there is certainly no angle formed at this point, and it is evident that the change from the level of 1 to that of 2 and 3 must be gradual, — must be, in fact, a regular motion which produces in the eye the effect of a curve ; but the mind reads this curve in the eye as the picture of a straight line, and refuses to think of a straight line, when the three drawings, Figs. 29, 30, and 31, are looked at as one picture.

It is difficult to believe that straight lines appear curved, but this appearance is always given by long straight lines which the mind does not know to be straight. At sunset the shadows of the clouds extend in straight lines, which are often practically horizontal with reference to any observer. These shadows appear as bands of dark, separated by the bright bands of the unobscured rays of sunlight, and both dark and light bands are seen radiating·from the sun, and becoming wider and wider as they recede from it and approach the spectator. Sometimes these cloud shadows may be seen extending to directly overhead, and sometimes they extend beyond the spectator toward the east, when they seem to converge opposite the sun, as they do in the west at the sun. When the impression of these lines extending from overhead toward both the west and the east is received, the effect of curvature is realized, for the mind does not think of these bands of light and dark as bounded by straight lines. The pupil may never be conscious of seeing the effect of curvature produced by straight lines. He may reason that, if he looks over the edge of a ruler, held horizontal, and in front of the line 2–1–3, that the edge of the ruler appears to coincide with the line, and thus the line must appear straight; but a short line near the eye will appear to cover a distant line which is miles long, and the ends of the ruler are relatively as much farther from the centre of the ruler as the points 2 and 3 are from point 1. Therefore, the ruler really causes in the eye the same curved line that the line 2–1–3 in the distance does.

If we study the eye, it is evident that all its images are upon a spherical surface, and so all lines upon this surface must be curved, whether they represent — that is, are pictured by — straight lines or curved lines. In the case of three vertical lines, represented by the points *A, C, B,* Fig. 17, one being directly in front and the others at the sides, three vertical planes composed of the visual rays are formed. The vertical planes formed by the rays to the central line *C* intersect the eye in a curve, which, in the top view, Fig. 17, is represented by *VC'*. The vertical planes formed by the rays to the lines at the sides, intersect the eye in curves, which, in Fig. 17, are represented by the lines *VB'* and *VA'*, and it is evident that the intersections of these three planes with the eye, must be curves which tend to intersect each other at two opposite points, represented in Fig. 17 by *V*, one being at the top of the eye and the other at the bottom. It is, how-

ever, not of the slightest consequence whether straight lines appear curved or not, for if the artist draws the different parts of the same straight lines, or of parallel straight lines as he sees them, the drawing resulting will give the effect of curvature. This is illustrated by Fig. 33, which reproduces the main lines of a published drawing by an artist who

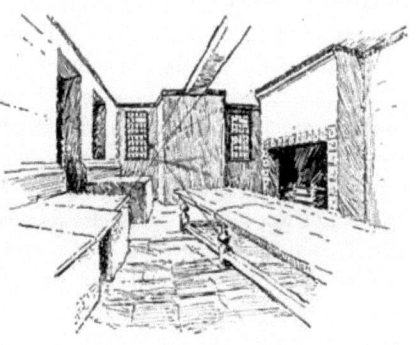

FIG. 33.   Incorrect Drawing.

drew just what he saw, without considering the effect thus produced, or the perspective principles which the artist must understand and apply. This drawing is similar in its errors to those which may often be found in the illustrations of our books and papers. These errors are due to the fact that the visual angles, in a subject causing large visual angles, are measured on so large a part of the surface of a sphere, that they cannot be approximately represented on the surface of a plane. In other words, we see in a sphere and draw on a plane; and, as the surface of the sphere cannot be developed, we cannot represent the different objects included in a subject causing large visual angles, so that the actual appearance of each object shall be given, and also the relations of the objects to each other. In the work of the artist, then, the least important must give way to the more important. To the pupil and the teacher it is more important that a correct impression of the whole, and of the relations of its parts, be given, than that the parts be true pictures and the impression of the whole be faulty; and thus it is often necessary for the artist to make the scientific perspective drawings which have been shown to be so false in representing the appearance of single objects.

Fig. 34 is a perspective drawing of four cubes whose vertical faces are in two vertical planes, parallel to the picture plane. When naturally seen, this drawing does not give the appearance which any one cube presents to the eye at the station-point, but it does give the impression of four equal cubes, and of the facts of their positions, and it is the best drawing that can be made of the four cubes thus placed. If the drawing is viewed from a point opposite *CV*, and about 4″ from the paper, the drawing of each cube will be foreshortened so as to create the same image in the eye as the cube it represents, but if the drawing is not thus seen, it is still the best drawing of the subject. The drawing is on a vertical picture plane, at right angles to the general direction in which the group of cubes is seen, and it illustrates the fact that when an object or a group of objects causing large visual angles is to be represented, a vertical picture plane, at right angles to a line to the centre of the group or the subject, must be used if the drawing is to give an idea of the facts of position and be satisfactory.

This is shown again by Figs. 35, 36, and 37. Fig. 35 is a perspective of a bureau, taken so as to give the appearance of inclination, which the horizontal lines of the drawer at the left must appear to have according to Rules 6 and 9. Fig. 36 is a perspective which, in the same way, gives the appearance of the drawer at the right. The left half of Fig. 35 is satisfactory if the right half is covered with paper, and the right half of Fig 36 is satisfactory if the left half is covered; but neither drawing gives a satisfactory impression of the whole bureau. To do this the perspective, Fig. 37, must be made on a plane at right angles to a horizontal line from the eye to a point over the centre of the bureau. These drawings illustrate the point shown also by Figs. 32 and 34, that the picture plane must

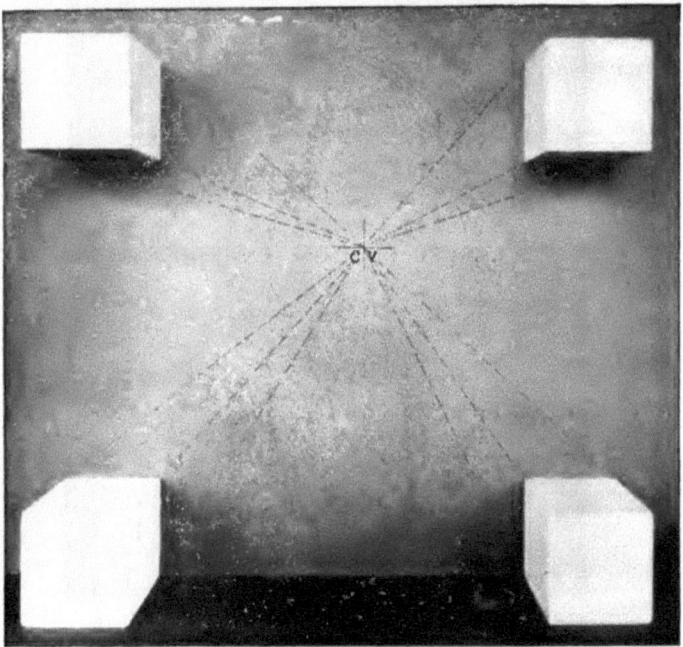

FIG. 34.   Scientific Perspective (Parallel).

be parallel to parallel straight lines which extend on both sides of the spectator if they are to be satisfactorily represented.

The station-point for Fig. 35 is about $3\frac{1}{2}''$ from the paper and opposite a point near the top of the cut and over the left drawer. If seen from this point, the drawing is foreshortened by having its left side nearer the eye than its right, and will not appear distorted.

The station-point for Fig. 36 is about $3\frac{1}{2}''$ from the paper and opposite a point near the top of the cut and over the right drawer. If seen from this point, the drawing is foreshortened by

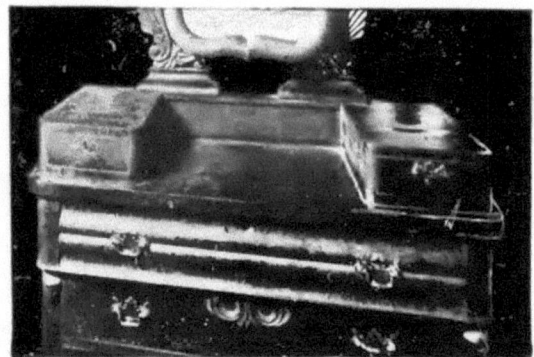

FIG. 35.   Gives Actual Appearance of the Drawer at the Left.

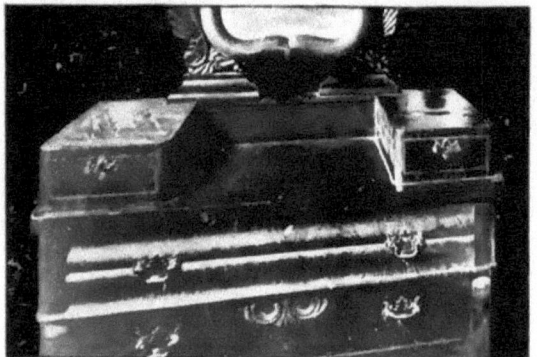

FIG. 36.   Gives Actual Appearance of the Drawer at the Right.

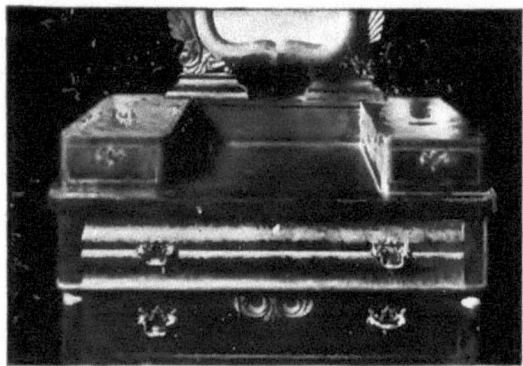

FIG. 37.   The Most Satisfactory Representation of the Whole.

having its right side nearer the eye than its left, and will not appear distorted.

We find that the artist draws single objects just as he sees them, or, rather, feels them, and that these drawings are generally satisfactory; but sometimes single objects cannot be represented satisfactorily just as they appear.

Fig. 38 is a perspective taken upon a vertical plane perpendicular to a line from the eye to a point just over the centre of the object. It is not a satisfactory drawing of a right prism, for it gives the idea of a block whose nearer end is not at right angles to the long edges.

Fig. 39 is a perspective drawing upon a plane parallel to the long edges, and is much more satisfactory than Fig. 38, although most of Fig. 38 is like the appearance, and most of Fig. 39 is unlike the appearance. If a piece of paper is held to cover the left-hand line of Fig. 38, the rest of the drawing will be satisfactory, while in Fig. 39 the larger part is different from what the eye sees, but necessarily so in order that the effect of an oblique prism is not produced.

If pupils have a single object to draw, and one end appears a vertical line, as in Fig. 38, they should, if possible, move so that this end becomes visible, and the drawing, Fig. 40, a satisfactory representation of the object, or so that the eye is between the two ends of the object, in which case the long lines would, as previously explained, be represented by horizontal lines, as in Figs. 32, 34, and 37. These drawings illustrate the following rules:

Rule 31. Whenever a vertical surface of a horizontal object is seen edgewise and appears a vertical line, any horizontal lines perpendicular to this surface must be represented by parallel horizontal lines.

Rule 32. Parallel horizontal lines connecting two vertical parallel surfaces, one at the right and the other at the left, must be represented by parallel horizontal lines; that is, when only one of the vertical faces of a horizontal prism is visible from any point between the ends of this surface, the horizontal lines of this and parallel surfaces must be represented by horizontal lines.

Rule 33. When any two vertical surfaces at right angles to each other are visible as surfaces at the same time, the horizontal lines of both must appear to vanish.

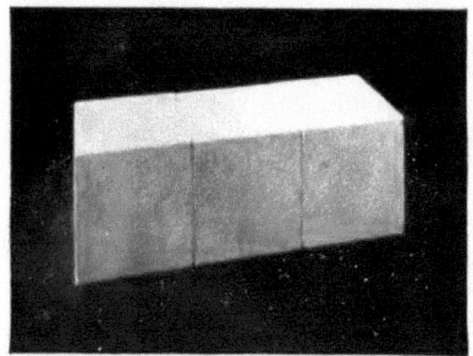

FIG.38.　An Unsatisfactory Drawing.

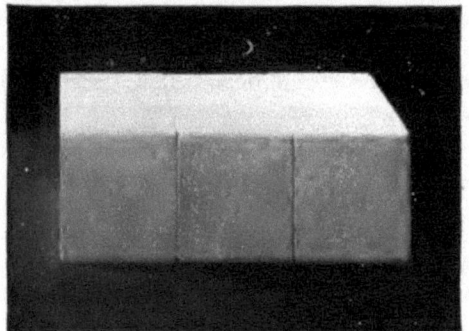

FIG. 39.　A Satisfactory Drawing.

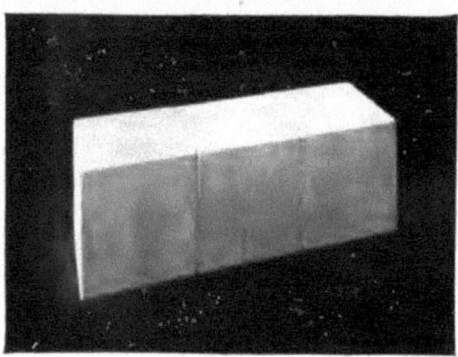

FIG. 40.　Satisfactory.

Rule 34. Any drawing representing by the use of two vanishing points, two systems of lines at right angles to each other, must always be placed between the two vanishing points.

Rule 35. Any drawing representing by the use of two vanishing points, two systems of lines at right angles to each other, and which extends to or beyond either vanishing point, must be distorted.

INTERIORS AND EXTERIORS.

The principles explained above should govern the representation of any subject of a geometric nature, without regard to the size of the subject, which is of no consequence, as the only point to be

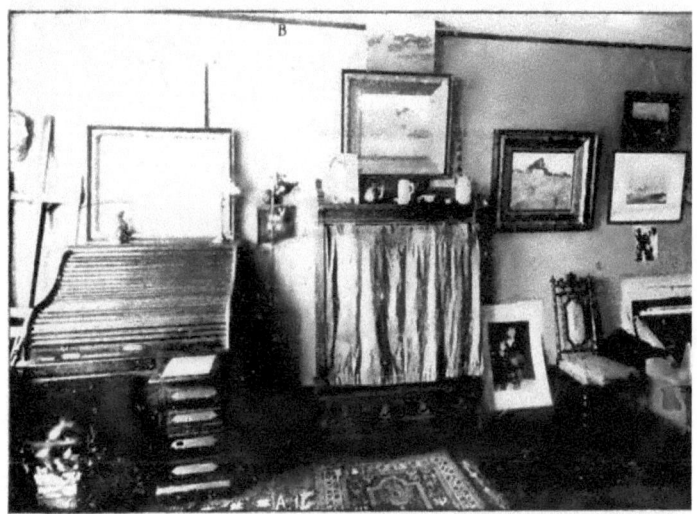

Fig. 41. A Serious Distortion of All at the Left of *A B*.

considered is the visual angle formed by the subject; but to show how the rules apply to interiors and exteriors, the following illustrations are given.

Fig. 41 is a perspective representing one wall of a room which vanishes to the right. The lines perpendicular to the wall vanish at point *CV* in *AB*; therefore, the drawing is unsatisfactory, for all

at the left of *AB* is outside of both vanishing points, and most
unpleasantly distorted. Fig. 36 shows the same distortion in the
left part of the bureau. The station-point from which Fig. 41 will
not appear distorted is about 2⅞" from *CV.*

If this wall is to be represented by converging lines, the station-
point must be about opposite the end of the room, and nothing at the

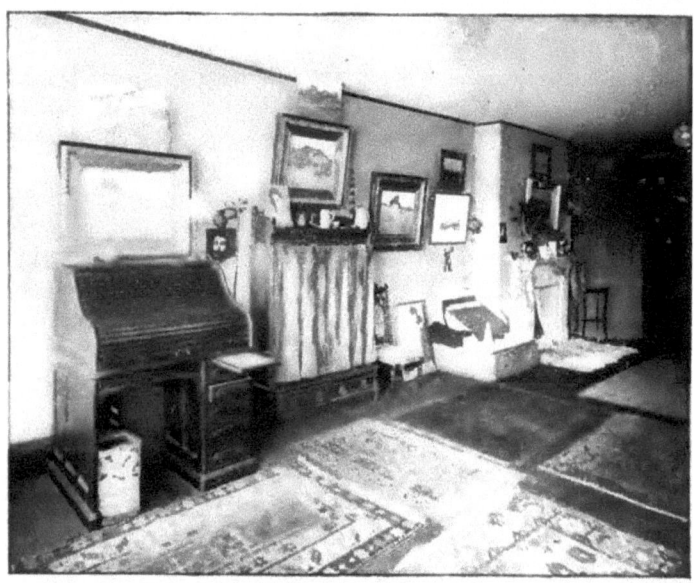

FIG. 42. A Satisfactory Representation of One Wall.

left of the left vanishing point can be shown. Fig. 42 represents
the wall when thus seen and is a satisfactory drawing. Like any
perspective it requires, however, to produce the same image as the
object, to be seen from the station-point, which is about 2⅞" from
the centre of the picture. When viewed naturally the perspective is
unpleasant though not distorted as in Fig. 41.

The wall may be represented as seen from a station-point about
opposite the centre of the wall. The resulting drawing, Fig. 43, is
satisfactory, though, as already shown, it does not represent the

appearance of the objects in the room unless the eye is at the station-point, which, in Fig. 43, is about 3″ from the paper, and opposite point *CV*. It gives, however, the positions of the objects with reference to the wall, and is often the best representation that can be made.

Fig. 44 represents two walls of a room as they are often illustrated. The drawing is unsatisfactory because it distorts the objects at the

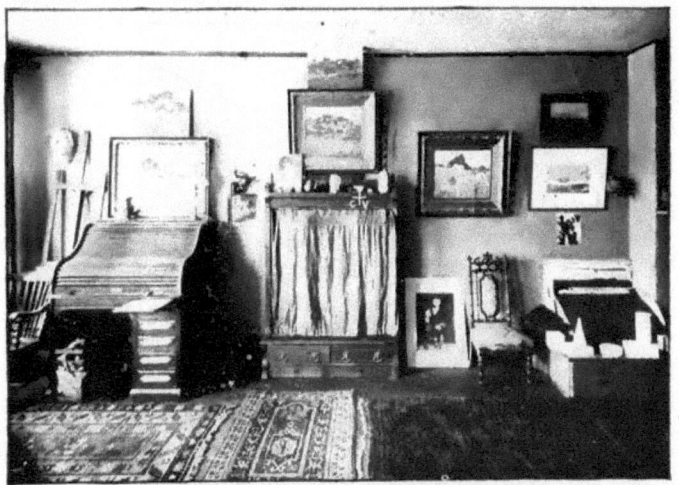

FIG. 43. A Satisfactory Representation of One Wall.

centre of the picture. The station-point for this drawing is about 3½″ from *CV*. There is no reason why these objects should be distorted, and if the picture plane is placed at right angles to a horizontal line from the eye to the centre of the subject, both walls will be at angles to the picture plane and their lines will vanish as in Fig. 45. The station-point for Fig. 45 is about 3½″ from the centre of the picture, and this figure illustrates the following rule:

Rule 36. When two walls of a room are to be represented about equally, the drawing should have two vanishing points for the horizontal lines of the walls and lines parallel to the walls.

Fig 46 represents three walls of a room, the picture plane being at right angles to a line from the eye to the centre of the subject. As the eye is nearer the wall at the left than that at the right, the horizontal lines of the end of the room are at an angle to the picture plane, and vanish to the right. The lines of the other walls vanish at point *CV* in *AB*, and the drawing is very unsatisfactory, for all at the left of *AB* is distorted. If Fig. 46 is viewed from a station-

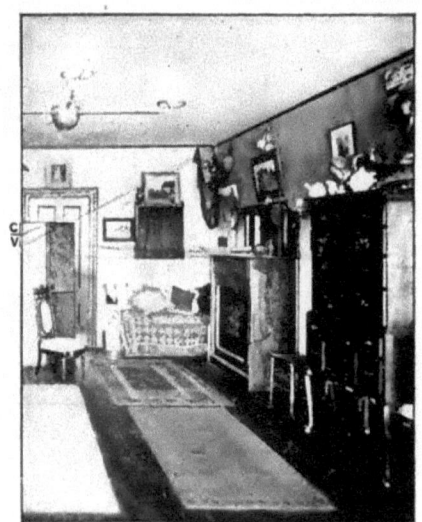

FIG. 44. An Unsatisfactory Drawing.

point opposite *CV* and about 3″ from the paper it will not appear distorted.

Fig. 47 is a perspective drawing on a plane parallel to the end of the room. It is the best drawing that can be made, and illustrates Rule 32 ; its station-point is about 3″ from the centre of the picture.

In drawing interiors the artist will generally represent the actual visual proportions of his subject as far as this can be done by representing straight lines by straight lines, but he will always give the actual appearance of separate objects and details of the subject, unless it is necessary to show the positions of these objects with reference to the principal lines of the room. When furniture or other details have their lines parallel to those of the walls, the artist is obliged to make practically the exact parallel perspective drawing illustrated by Figs. 34, 37, 43, and 47. The artist may sometimes depart from the proportions of these parallel perspective drawings and give the foreshortening seen in horizontal and vertical

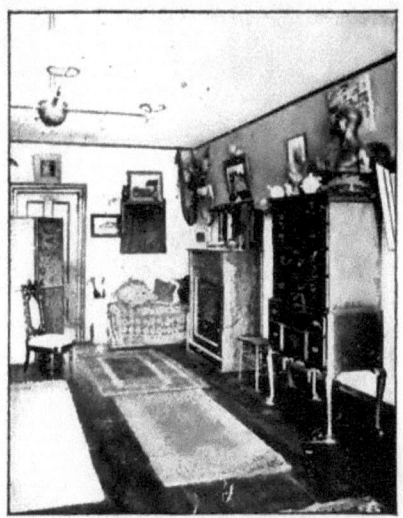

FIG. 45. A Satisfactory Drawing.

dimensions, but when subjects similar to those mentioned above are to be represented, it is generally best to make the exact perspective drawing which requires to be seen from one fixed point.

This is true, however, only with regard to geometric subjects, for the artist always represents other subjects just as he sees them. In figure drawing, for instance, he draws each figure just as he sees it, and would never think of making a scientific perspective drawing of such a subject as the Lord's Supper, except as regards the room.

Fig. 48 is a top view representing the station-point or eye of a spectator who stands in front of the central cylinder, *B*, of a row of

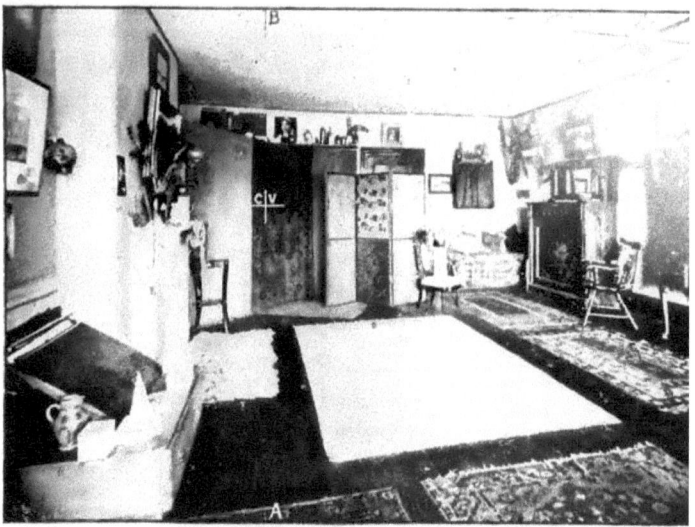

Fig. 46. A Serious Distortion of all at the Left of *A B.*

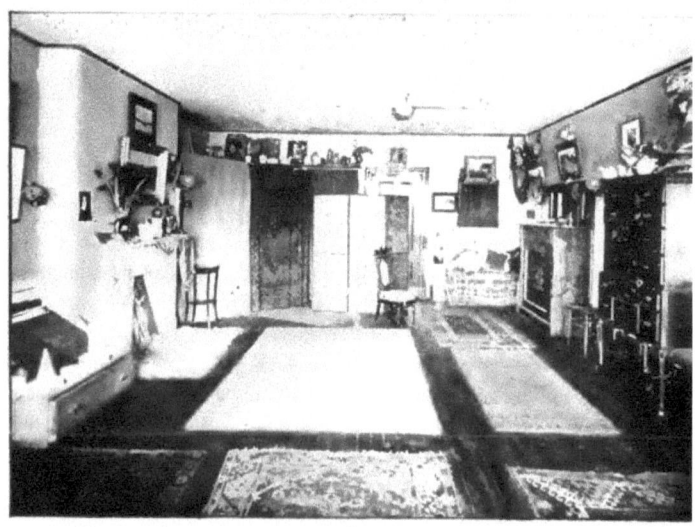

Fig. 47. A Satisfactory Representation.

three equal cylinders, *A, B;* and *C,* and traces upon a vertical
picture plane placed against the cylinders lines to cover each
cylinder and form the perspective of the cylinders; the cylinders
may roughly represent three equal figures. The visual rays from *A*
and *B* to the station-point pass through the picture plane obliquely,
and thus the widths 3–4 and 5–6 of the drawings of *A* and *C* are
wider than 1–2 which represents the central figure. To make a

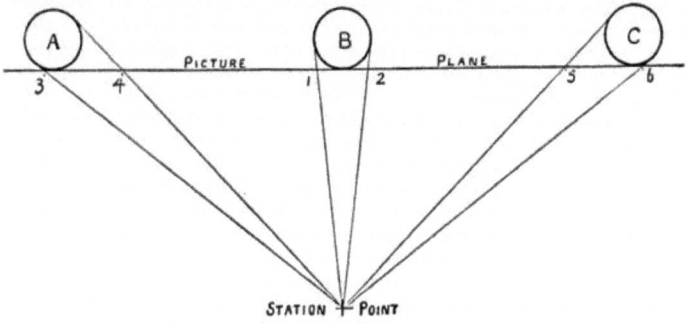

FIG. 48. A Top View.

scientific perspective, then, of figures arranged as in the Lord's
Supper, the figures at the extremes of the canvas should be represented as much stouter or wider than those at the centre, in order
that they will appear the same size as those at the centre when they
are foreshortened by being seen obliquely by the eye situated at the
station-point; and this no artist would think of doing, for he always
draws what he sees, and represents each figure so that it will look
right when seen from a point directly in front of it.

When drawing exteriors and outdoor subjects, the principles
governing the representation of objects and interiors should, with
few exceptions, be applied. If the eye is opposite or very near one
end or side of a large building of which one side only is seen, this
side may be represented by vanishing lines, as in Fig. 42, but never
so as to distort, as Fig. 41 distorts the desk. If the eye is situated
as in Fig. 41, or is near the centre of the side to be represented, the
horizontal lines of the side must be represented by horizontal lines,

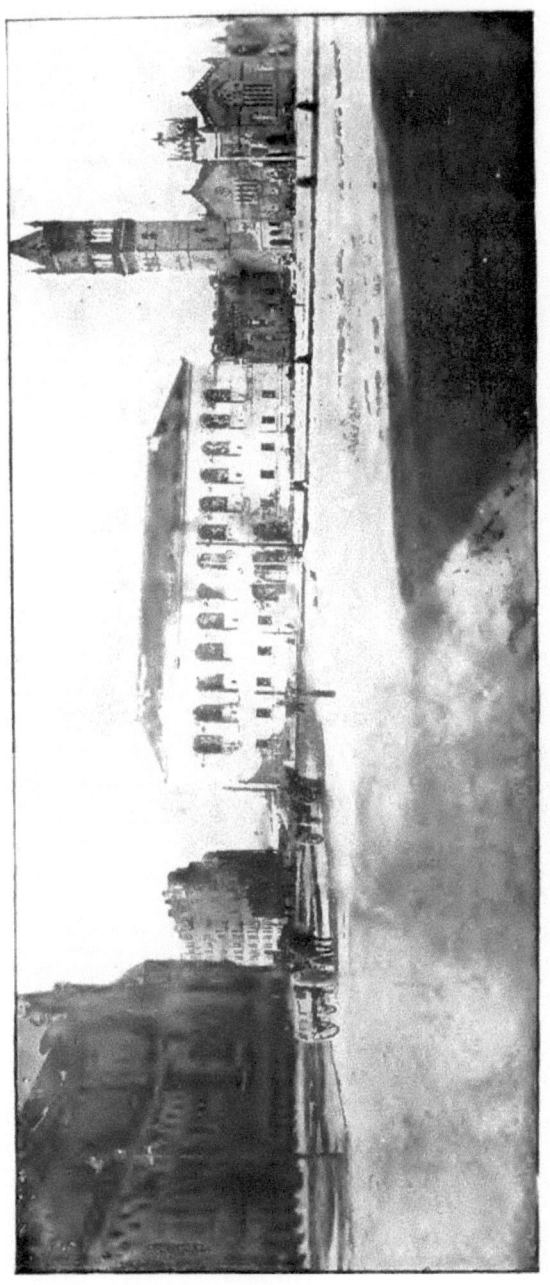

FIG. 50. A Panoramic Photograph. It is a Curvilinear Perspective and represents Straight Lines by Curves

as in Fig. 43. If two vertical sides of a rectangular building are seen, the horizontal lines of both must vanish.

When drawing a landscape, the artist will represent just what he sees and obtain a satisfactory picture, unless there are long straight lines, or straight lines causing large visual angles in the subject. In this case, if the artist draws what he sees, he will, as already shown, represent the straight lines by curved lines, and generally produce an unsatisfactory drawing.

In drawing an ordinary landscape or street scene, if the artist draws just what he sees, as he looks at the different parts of the subject, he is really making a drawing upon what is practically the vertical surface of a hollow cylinder; for his subject has so little height in comparison with its width, that a vertical picture plane at right angles to the direction in which any part is seen will give practically a true picture of this part. As the artist turns, this vertical picture plane will sweep through a cylindrical surface, and an artist's drawing of an outdoor subject taking in a wide visual angle is practically the development of the surface of the cylinder upon which true pictures of the different parts are obtained. A drawing upon a cylindrical surface is called a cylindrical perspective, and represents parallel straight lines by curved lines which converge at opposite points.

A drawing which represents straight lines by curves is generally unsatisfactory. In some cases it may not be objectionable, and drawings of this nature have been made by noted artists. The student should never be allowed to make such a drawing, and the artist should do so only when the straight lines are frequently broken, or in different planes, so that it is not evident, at first glance, that the lines are straight and parallel. The same effect of curvature is produced by long vertical lines as by long parallel horizontal lines; the artist may represent this convergence in the verticals, though not as often as he may represent the curvature of horizontal lines.

Fig. 49 is a curvilinear perspective which was taken with a revolving camera upon a cylindrical negative. It represents the Boston Public Library, with the Art Museum at the left and the New Old South Church at the right.

Fig. 50 represents the same subject by a common plane perspective drawing, which gives the idea of a straight street. From Fig. 49 we get the idea of a curved street and building. Fig. 50 is far preferable, and the artist should always represent straight lines by straight lines, unless the conditions are such that the effect of curvature is not noticeable or unpleasant; but this is a question for the artist, the teacher and student should always represent straight lines by straight lines.

Although Fig. 50 is preferable to Fig. 49, it distorts the parts at the right and left very unpleasantly, and the artist who wishes to represent the Library should omit the Art Museum, so as to be able to represent the Library and Church as they appear and by the use of two vanishing points. Fig. 51 shows how the artist may combine the horizontal dimensions of the curvilinear perspective, Fig. 49, with the straight lines of a plane perspective to produce the most satisfactory representation of the subject.

It is evident that any drawing, whether a scientific or a free-hand perspective, should be seen from a certain distance and point in order to produce the best effect. In drawings of single objects this point is generally outside the scientific perspective, so that the drawing is distorted when it is seen naturally. Of course, a free-hand perspective may be distorted by being seen obliquely; but drawings are naturally viewed perpendicularly, so that it requires an effort to view a free-hand perspective incorrectly, while the effort is required to see the scientific perspective correctly.

The free-hand perspective causes practically the same image in the eye whatever the distance be from which it is viewed, and when it is not seen from the proper station-point the impression received from it differs from that received from the objects only in regard to the relative sizes of the objects it represents. When a scientific perspective is not seen from its station-point there is not only this change in the relative sizes of the objects, but also changes in their appearances; so every consideration favors the use of the free-hand perspective instead of the scientific.

It has been shown that the artist's drawing is not a drawing which can be made upon any plane, whatever its position. Another point of difference between the artist's drawing and any perspective is due to the fact that a perspective represents what is seen by one eye, or from one fixed point, while the artist's drawing represents the facts of form realized by means of two eyes, that is, two station-points. The difference between a perspective and what is seen with both eyes will be readily appreciated by looking at any subject containing objects at different distances, first with one eye, then with the other, and then with both at once. By means of our two eyes we appreciate the roundness or solidity of objects and also their distances apart. These are the qualities which are most important to the artist, and it will be readily seen that his drawing must be a matter of feeling and not of science.

The pupil who uses the glass slate, except in work from copies, must close one eye to test accurately, and his drawing is thus a perspective. But this work is elementary, and necessary to prepare the pupil to see accurately enough to draw with feeling in later work when the slate is not used, and it gives the best preparatory education that can be obtained.

We must decide that the teacher should adopt the artist's methods, and enable pupils to draw first what the eye sees, — that is, what will give the best impression of the appearance and the facts of single objects or subjects causing small visual angles, — and then to teach them to apply perspective principles, as they may be needed to correct the drawings made by eye from geometric subjects causing wide visual angles, and finally to teach them the principles of scientific perspective, so that when this drawing is required, as it often will be, they may be able to produce it. But the teacher or student of perspective is not wise to insist that the artist shall always make scientific perspective drawings; for he does not do this, and never will in his highest work, and we must accept the uniform practice of all great artists of the past and present to decide the point that it is not best to make, unless compelled to, a scientific perspective drawing which requires to be seen from one fixed point.

SUMMARY.

Drawings may be arranged in the following classes:

1. Drawings representing the appearance of a single object whose position is of no consequence.

2. Drawings representing the appearance and the position of a single object.

3. Drawings representing more than one object, and giving the impression of their appearances and their relations.

In the first class may be placed drawings of crystals, insects, foliage, and similar subjects whose form and construction or color are to be represented. The question of the picture plane is simple in all such cases; for, as the object may occupy any position, we may represent its actual appearance upon a plane inclined in any position, so as to be at right angles to the direction in which the object is seen, and a satisfactory picture will result. Such drawings are generally made to show the facts of the object as far as possible, and are scientific rather than artistic; and the object would be placed so as to present these facts, which would then be represented upon a plane which would often be parallel to the principal face or surface of the object.

The second class includes all illustrative and artistic work.

It has been shown that the picture which, when viewed naturally, produces an image in the eye like that which the object would produce must be, if upon a plane, on one which is perpendicular to the central visual ray. But we have seen that a picture on an inclined picture plane is not satisfactory, and that the drawing which the artist makes always represents vertical lines by vertical lines, and that in effect it is practically what is given by drawing on a vertical picture plane and giving the visual proportions instead of the elongated drawing which a vertical plane produces when an object is above or below the level of the eye, so that the visual rays pass through it obliquely.

As the artist's work generally represents objects near the eye level, or extending about equally below and above it, and not causing very large visual angles, we may say that, practically, he makes use of a vertical picture plane perpendicular to the central visual ray.

If an exact drawing on any plane is to be made, it must be that on a vertical picture plane; but it is not necessary that the young pupil consider the question of the picture plane, for he should be taught to draw what he sees, except when representing vertical lines which appear to converge, and objects placed so as to appear like

Fig. 38. If he uses the slate to determine the proportions of an object, he should hold it at right angles to the direction in which he sees the object, and should change the drawing, when it represents vertical lines by inclined lines, by substituting vertical for the inclined lines. He should measure proportions by the pencil in the same way, holding it at right angles to the direction in which he sees the object. Practically, objects are generally so little above or below the eye level, that the question of the inclination of the plane is of little consequence to the draughtsman and advanced pupil. If pupils draw upon the slate from objects near them, and are too young to understand how to change the drawing by representing the vertical edges by vertical lines, it will be better for them to make the exact picture or tracing, until old enough to change it, than to obtain the idea that they see what is given on a vertical picture plane; but it is not necessary for pupils to think of the picture plane even when the slate is used, and teachers should enable pupils to draw first and theorize afterwards.

The third class includes all pictures representing several objects and a large visual angle.

A vertical picture plane at right angles to the central visual ray should be used for such subjects; but instead of making the exact perspective drawing of small objects and details away from the centre of the picture, so that these objects are distorted unless they are foreshortened by being seen obliquely, it is better to represent them just as they appear when it is not necessary to show their relative positions. Thus the circles of plinth B, Fig. 24, appear horizontal ellipses, and there is no reason why the representation of plinth B should not be exactly like that of plinth A. The cube at the right of Fig. 41 is distorted, for the eye sees the two outer corners of the top face on the same level, and they should be so represented when it is not necessary to show that the edges of the cube are parallel to those of the box upon which it rests. The cone at the right of the cube can be represented by the horizontal ellipse which the eye sees, unless it is tangent to a square (or other figure) which is situated and represented as is the top of either lower cube in Fig. 33; in this case it may be necessary, in order to show that the circle is tangent to the square, to represent it by an inclined ellipse. In the same way the objects at the right of Fig. 43 may be represented as they appear, and any object situated as is the pitcher or the plinth in Fig. 46, and bounded by horizontal circles, should always be represented as it appears. The objects in the lower left part of Fig. 47 are not distorted as much as they are in Fig. 46, but always in any perspective representation for artistic purposes single detached objects should be represented just as they appear, unless it is necessary to show their relations to other parts of the subject.

Often, however, it will be necessary to represent objects by the use of one vanishing point at the level of the eye, and the exact parallel perspective on the vertical picture plane is the most satisfactory representation of many geometric subjects. The pupil may obtain, when sketching from nature, the proportions of such a drawing by measuring with the pencil held parallel to the front faces of the objects instead of at right angles to the directions in which they are seen. The simplest and surest test would be the use of the slate held vertical and parallel to the front faces of the objects.

NOTE. — The photographs from which Figs. 49 and 50 were made have been copyrighted by N. L. Stebbins, 132 Boylston St., Boston. Copies will be printed to order by him.

CHAPTER VIII.

COMPOSITION.

COMPOSITION means the arrangement of parts to produce a whole, and is good when the effect produced is harmonious and pleasing. Composition is a subject which, according to the views of most artists, cannot be taught. Certainly the beauty and pleasure which are due to the arrangements produced by a master cannot be derived from any formal application of principles, derived from study of the master's work; and those without genius can only hope to produce work which does not violate the common rules of good taste.

This is a subject with which little can be done in the public schools, but those interested in it will do well to read John Burnet's book on painting, and "Elements of Drawing," by Ruskin. From the latter book, the following extracts are taken :

" Composition means, literally and simply, putting several things together, so as to make *one* thing out of them ; the nature and goodness of which they have all a share in producing. Thus a musician composes an air, by putting notes together in certain relations ; a poet composes a poem by putting thoughts and words in pleasant order ; and a painter a picture, by putting thoughts, forms, and colors in pleasant order."

" In all these cases, observe, an intended unity must be the result of composition. A paver cannot be said to compose the heap of stones which he empties from his cart, nor the sower the handful of seed which he scatters from his hand. It is the essence of composition that everything should be in a determined place, perform an intended part, and act, in that part, advantageously for everything that is connected with it. . . .

" In a well-composed air, no note, however short or low, can be spared. . . . In a good poem, each word and thought enhances the value of those which precede and follow it ; and every syllable has a loveliness which depends not so much on its abstract sound as on its position."

" Much more in a great picture ; every line and color is so arranged as to advantage the rest. None are inessential, however slight ; and none are independent, however forcible. It is not enough that they truly represent natural objects, but they must fit into certain places, and gather in certain harmonious groups; so that, for instance, the red chimney of a cottage is not merely set in its place as a chimney, but that it may affect, in a certain way pleasurable to the eye, the pieces of green or blue in other parts of the picture; and we ought to see that the work is masterly, merely by the positions and quantities of these patches of green, red, and blue, even at a distance which renders it perfectly impossible to determine what the colors represent, or to see whether the red is a chimney or an old woman's cloak, and whether the blue is smoke, sky, or water."

"It seems to be appointed, in order to remind us, in all we do, of the great laws of Divine government and human polity, that composition in the arts should strongly affect every order of mind, however unlearned or thoughtless. Hence the popular delight in rhythm and metre, and in simple musical melodies. But it is also appointed that *power* of composition in the fine arts should be an exclusive attribute of great intellect. All men can more or less copy what they see, and, more or less, remember it. . . . But the gift of composition is not given *at all* to more than one man in a thousand; in its highest range, it does not occur above three or four times in a century."

"It follows, from these general truths, that it is impossible to give rules which will enable you to compose. You might much more easily receive rules to enable you to be witty. If it were possible to be witty by rule, wit would cease to be either admirable or amusing; if it were possible to compose melody by rule, Mozart and Cimarosa need not have been born; if it were possible to compose pictures by rule, Titian and Veronese would be ordinary men. The essence of composition lies precisely in the fact of its being unteachable, in its being the operation of an individual mind of range and power exalted above others."

"But though no one can *invent* by rule, there are some simple laws of arrangement which it is well for you to know, because, though they will not enable you to produce a good picture, they will often assist you to set forth what goodness may be in your work in a more telling way than you could have done otherwise; and, by tracing them in the work of good composers, you may better understand the grasp of their imagination, and the power it possesses over their materials."

Mr. Ruskin states the following to be the chief laws governing composition:

First.   "The Law of Principality."
Second. "The Law of Repetition."
Third.   "The Law of Continuity."

Fourth. " The Law of Curvature."
Fifth. " The Law of Radiation."
Sixth. " The Law of Contrast."
Seventh. " The Law of Interchange."
Eighth. " The Law of Consistency."
Ninth. " The Law of Harmony."

" The Law of Principality " deals with the unity of the composition ; " that is, to make out of many things one whole ; the first mode in which this can be effected is, by determining that *one* feature shall be more important than the rest, and that the others shall group with it."

" The Law of Repetition " concerns the expression of " sympathy among the different objects, and perhaps the pleasantest, because most surprising, kind of sympathy, is when one group imitates or repeats another ; not in the way of balance or symmetry, but subordinately, like a far-away and broken echo of it. . . .

" Symmetry, or the balance of parts or masses in nearly equal opposition, is one of the conditions of treatment under the law of Repetition. . . .

" Symmetry in Nature is, however, never formal nor accurate. She takes the greatest care to secure some difference between the corresponding things or parts of things ; and an approximation to accurate symmetry is only permitted in animals because their motions secure perpetual difference between the balancing parts. . . .

" The Law of Continuity " concerns the " pleasurable way of expressing unity by giving some orderly succession to a number of objects more or less similar. And this succession is most interesting when it is connected with some gradual change in the aspect or character of the objects. . . . If there be no change at all in the shape or size of the objects, there is no continuity ; there is only repetition — monotony."

" The Law of Curvature " is the law of beauty. " All beautiful objects whatsoever are terminated by delicately curved lines, except where the straight line is indispensable to their use or stability. . . .

" As curves are more beautiful than straight lines, it is necessary to a good composition that its continuities of object, mass, or color should be, if possible, in curves, rather than straight lines or angular ones. . . .

" The Law of Radiation " enforces unison of action in arising from, or proceeding to, some given point. It treats of the harmonious grouping of lines which spring from or are directed to a single point.

" The Law of Contrast." " Of course, the character of everything is best manifested by Contrast. Rest can only be enjoyed after labor ; sound, to be heard clearly, must rise out of silence ; light is exhibited by darkness,

darkness by light ; and so on in all things.   Now in art every color has an opponent color, which, if brought near it, will relieve it more completely than any other ; so, also, every form and line may be made more striking to the eye by an opponent form or line near them ; a curved line is set off by a straight one, a massy form by a slight one, and so on ; and in all good work, nearly double the value, which any given color or form would have uncombined, is given to each by contrast.

"In this case again, however, a too manifest use of the artifice vulgarizes a picture.   Great painters do not commonly, or very visibly, admit violent contrast.   They introduce it by stealth and with intermediate links of tender change ; allowing, indeed, the opposition to tell upon the mind as a surprise, but not as a shock."

"The Law of Interchange" concerns the alternation of light and dark and color, by means of which the unity of opposite things is enforced, by giving to each a portion of the character of the other.

"One of the most curious facts which will impress itself upon you, when you have drawn some time carefully from Nature in light and shade, is the appearance of intentional artifice with which contrasts of this alternate kind are produced by her ; the artistry with which she will darken a tree trunk as long as it comes against light sky, and throw sunlight on it precisely at the spot where it comes against a dark hill, and similarly treat all her masses of shade and color, is so great, that if you only follow her closely, every one who looks at your drawing with attention will think that you have been inventing the most artificially and unnaturally delightful interchange of shadow that could possibly be devised by human wit."[1]

"The Law of Consistency" bears principally "on the separate masses or divisions of a picture : the character of the whole composition may be broken or various, if we please, but there must certainly be a tendency to consistent assemblage in its divisions.   As an army may act on several points at once, but can only act effectually by having somewhere formed and regular masses, and not wholly by skirmishers ; so a picture may be various in its tendencies, but must be somewhere united and coherent in its masses.   Good composers are always associating their colors in great groups ; binding their forms together by encompassing lines, and securing, by various dexterities of expedient, what they themselves call 'breadth': that is to say, a large gathering of each kind of thing into one place ; light being gathered to light, darkness to darkness, and color to color.   If, however, this be done by introducing false lights or false colors, it is absurd

[1] This sentence probably means that those not students of nature will think true studies "artificial and unnatural."

and monstrous; the skill of a painter consists in obtaining breadth by rational arrangement of his objects, not by forced or wanton treatment of them. . . . Generally speaking, however, breadth will result in sufficient degree from fidelity of study: Nature is always broad; and if you paint her colors in true relations, you will paint them in majestic masses. If you find your work look broken and scattered, it is, in all probability, not only ill composed, but untrue."

"The Law of Harmony." "There are all kinds of harmonies in a picture, according to its mode of production. There is even a harmony of touch. If you paint one part of it very rapidly and forcibly, and another part slowly and delicately, each division of the picture may be right separately, but they will not agree together: the whole will be effectless and valueless, out of harmony. Similarly, if you paint one part of it by a yellow light in a warm day, and another by a gray light in a cold day, though both may have been sunlight, and both may be well toned, and have their relative shadows truly cast, neither will look like light: they will destroy each other's power, by being out of harmony. These are only broad and definable instances of discordance; but there is an extent of harmony in all good work much too subtle for definition; depending on the draughtsman's carrying everything he draws up to just the balancing and harmonious point, in finish, and color, and depth of tone, and intensity of moral feeling, and style of touch, all considered at once; and never allowing himself to lean too emphatically on detached parts, or exalt one thing at the expense of another, or feel acutely in one place and coldly in another."

The chapter from which these notes are taken is most interesting. Throughout Ruskin's works there are the most valuable and modern ideas on art, in even its most recent phase of impressionism. It is difficult to reconcile these views, which have so recently become somewhat generally understood, with other statements by Ruskin, which are of an entirely different nature, and which, carried out, will tend to produce no more artistic work than the paintings done by Ruskin himself. Seeing these paintings, it is difficult to believe that the theories underlying the luminous and bright paintings of to-day are not due much more to Turner, who is admitted to be one of the first impressionists, than they are to Ruskin, who, as his friend, must have received from him inspiration for much that is good in his writings.

The following paragraphs on Composition are taken from John Burnet's book on Painting:

"Composition is the art of arranging figures or objects, so as to adapt them to any particular subject. In composition, four requisites are necessary :—that the story be well told ; that it possess a good general form ; that it be so arranged as to be capable of receiving a proper effect of light and shade ; and that it be susceptible of an agreeable disposition of color. The form of a composition is best suggested by the subject or design, as the fitness of the adaptation ought to appear to emanate from the circumstances themselves ; hence the variety of compositions.

"To secure a good general form in composition, it is necessary that it should be as simple as possible. A confused, complicated form may hide the art, but can never invite the attention. Whether this is to be produced by a breadth of light and shade, which is often the case with Rembrandt, even on a most complicated outline, or by the simple arrangement of color, as we often find in Titian or Raffaelle's works, must depend upon the state of the artist. It is sufficient to direct the younger students to this particular, their minds being generally carried away by notions of variety and contrast.

"As I have made use of the terms 'beautiful and agreeable arrangements,' it is proper to give an explanation of the sense in which they are applied. By a beautiful arrangement, I mean a proper adaptation of those principles that arrest a common observer, and give a pleasurable sensation, which to a cultivated mind increases (not diminishes) by the investigation of the cause which produces it. For example, a beautiful appearance in nature affects the savage and the philosopher from their sensations merely as men; but a painter, whose life is spent in a constant competition with nature in producing the same effects, receives a tenfold gratification in following her through those assemblages which to the world beside are, as it were, 'a fountain sealed and a book shut up.' Hence, in art, a beautiful arrangement must be a selection of those forms, lights, and colors that produce a similar result ; and the taste of an artist is shown in heightening their effect by the absence of those circumstances which are found by experience to produce the contrary. Did an investigation of the means pursued by the great masters tend to abridge an artist's pleasurable sensations, instead of being the most favored, he would be rendered the most miserable of beings; but the opposite is the case, as by such means he is taught an alphabet that enables him to understand the language of nature. It may be supposed, that in my search after so desirable an object, I have perused all the works written to define Beauty and Taste, and which endeavor to circumscribe with a line that endless variety and omnipresence which make nature a source of gratification to all natures under every alteration of the mind; but as I wish to avoid all controversy on the subject, which we often find merely renders the most sublime truths more obscure, I shall only remark that, as far as painting is concerned, the authors of many of these works have done an irreparable injury. Artists generally prefer the opinions of untutored children to the remarks of the most learned philosophers, whose advancement in other sciences really seems to increase their ignorance of this. If I have explained my definition of the terms sufficiently for the artist's comprehension, I am satisfied. To explain them to others, would be as equally impossible as that those others should define them to us. The mind must have received its education through the medium of the eye, not of the ear, to enjoy the faculty of conceiving such ideas, or the power of tracing them to their original source in nature, or in art, as a test of their truth."

The following paragraphs on Composition are taken from Sir Joshua Reynold's Work:

DISCOURSE VIII.

" To apply these general observations, which belong equally to all arts, to ours in particular. In a composition, when the objects are scattered and divided into many equal parts, the eye is perplexed and fatigued, from not knowing where to find the principal action, or which is the principal figure; for where all are making equal pretensions to notice, all are in equal danger of neglect.

"The expression which is used very often, on these occasions is, the piece wants repose; a word which perfectly expresses a relief of the mind from that state of hurry and anxiety which it suffers, when looking at a work of this character.

" On the other hand absolute unity, that is, a large work, consisting of one group or mass of light only, would be as defective as an heroic poem without episode, or any collateral incidents to recreate the mind with that variety which it always requires.

" It is given as a rule by Fresnoy, That *the principal figure of a subject must appear in the midst of the picture, under the principal light, to distinguish it from the rest.* A painter who should think himself obliged strictly to follow this rule, would encumber himself with needless difficulties; he would be confined to great uniformity of composition and be deprived of many beauties which are incompatible with its observance. The meaning of this rule extends, or ought to extend, no further than this: — That the principal figure should be immediately distinguished at the first glance of

the eye; but there is no necessity that the principal light should fall on the
principal figure, or that the principal figure should be in the middle of the
picture. It is sufficient that it be distinguished by its place, or by the
attention of other figures pointing it out to the spectator. So far is this
rule from being indispensable, that it is very seldom practiced, other con-
siderations of greater consequence often standing in the way. Examples in
opposition to this rule, are found in the Cartoons, in Christ's Charge to
Peter, the Preaching of St. Paul, and Elymas the Sorcerer, who is undoubt-
edly the principal object in that picture. In none of these compositions is
the principal figure in the middle of the picture. In the very admirable
composition of the Tent of Darius, by LeBrun, Alexander is not in the
middle of the picture, nor does the principal light fall on him; but the attention of all the other figures immediately distinguishes him, and distinguishes him more properly; the greatest light falls on the daughter of
Darius, who is in the middle of the picture, where it is more necessary the
principal light should be placed."

DISCOURSE III.

"Having gone thus far in our investigation of the great style in painting, — if we now should suppose that the artist has found the true idea of
beauty, which enables him to give his works a correct and perfect design, —
if we should suppose, also, that he has acquired a knowledge of the unadulter-
ated habits of Nature, which gives him simplicity, — the rest of his task is,
perhaps, less than is generally imagined. Beauty and simplicity have so great
a share in the composition of a great style, that he who has acquired them
has little else to learn. It must not, indeed, be forgotten, that there is a
nobleness of conception, which goes beyond anything in the mere exhibition
even of perfect form ; there is an art of animating and dignifying the figures
with intellectual grandeur, of impressing the appearance of philosophic
wisdom, or heroic virtue. This can only be acquired by him who enlarges
the sphere of his understanding by a variety of knowledge, and varies his
imagination with the best productions of ancient and modern poetry.

"A hand thus exercised, and a mind thus instructed, will bring the Art
to a higher degree of excellence than perhaps it has hitherto attained in this
country. Such a student will disdain the humbler walks of painting, which,
however profitable, can never assure him a permanent reputation. He will
leave the meaner Artist servilely to suppose that those are the best pictures
which are most likely to deceive the spectator. He will permit the lower
painter, like the florist or collector of shells, to exhibit the minute discrim-

inations, which distinguish one object of the same species from another; while he, like the philosopher, will consider Nature in the abstract, and represent in every one of his figures the character of its species.

"If deceiving the eye were the only business of the Art, there is no doubt, indeed, but the minute painter would be more apt to succeed; but it is not the eye, it is the mind which the painter of genius desires to address; nor will he waste a moment upon those smaller objects which only serve to catch the sense, to divide the attention, and to counteract his great design of speaking to the heart.

"This is the ambition which I wish to excite in your minds; and the object I have had in my view throughout this discourse, is that one great idea which gives to painting its true dignity, which entitles it to the name of a Liberal Art, and makes it a sister of poetry."

The preceding pages present the principles underlying the arrangement of a work of art. Those who wish to study the application of these principles should read Burnet's book, which is one of the most valuable, and covers all the subjects relating to painting.

The impossibility of teaching composition, and especially in the public schools, has been shown. Though little can be done, the subject should not be wholly neglected. The most valuable education in it will be given by study of the works of the best masters, which should be placed in every schoolroom where they can be seen by all the pupils. These works will exert an influence for good upon all.

The principles explained apply not only to the arrangement of pictures, but to the simple subjects which are suitable for study in the public schools; and a proper arrangement of these objects is so simple that the principles will be readily applied by those who are not artists, or trained to perceive the finest sensations.

The result of all study of this subject will be to enforce the necessity of simplicity and breadth in form, in light and shade, and in color. There must be a point of principal interest, a point to which all others are subordinate, and the drawing or picture must explain itself at a glance.

In the lower grades when pupils draw from a single object, they must place the drawing in a pleasing manner upon the paper, and make it the size which will produce the best effect. Many pupils will make a minute drawing, and place it in one corner of the sheet; others will make a drawing which extends to the edges of the paper, and often should go beyond the edge in one or two directions. But few will make the drawing the best size, or place it properly.

A common mistake is to place the drawing very near the lower edge of the paper. The effect produced by this is very unpleasant, for the drawing should have as much space below it as above, and often more. Without this space the perspective effect is destroyed. Teachers must insist that the blocking-in lines be drawn so as to give a drawing of the best size for the paper, and well placed upon it.

When two or more objects are placed together, there is the question of their choice and arrangement. From what has been said, it will be seen that objects which are entirely unrelated cannot be arranged to convey an idea. Objects should be arranged so as not to produce a scattered and spotty effect, and they should not be of the same size or shape; one object should be important through size, and color, and position. They should be arranged so as to avoid the monotony due to long and absolutely unbroken lines, and the principal object should not be placed exactly in the centre of the page. It is better to have simple backgrounds, to concentrate the objects and keep them one side of the centre, than to cover the background equally by the objects. An odd number of objects is better than an even, and they should be arranged so that there shall be one principal high light and at least two secondary lights in the group. The effect of light and dark must be simple and produced by masses of light in contrast with masses of dark. Groups should be arranged so that the foregrounds appear lighter than the backgrounds.

Burnet divides composition into two classes, angular and circular. In angular, the objects are arranged so that the important lines form a mass whose general shape is triangular. In circular, the important lines are circular or elliptical. A subject should always be composed so as to come under one class or the other. The angular form is the most simple for groups of still life, and is usually adopted for these subjects. The illustrations show the triangular form.

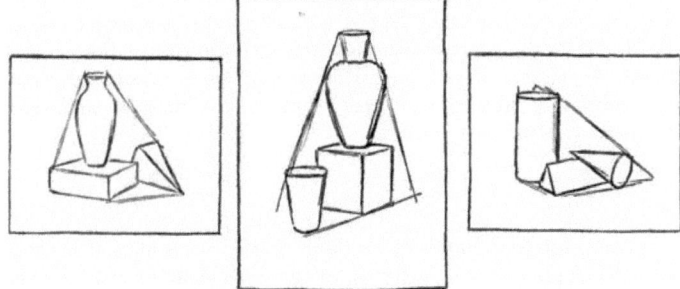

The following extracts from Sir Joshua Reynolds' *Discourses* are given on account of their special value in connection with the subject of this book and chapter :

DISCOURSE V.

"There is another caution which I wish to give you. Be as select in those whom you endeavor to please, as in those whom you endeavor to imitate. Without the love of fame, you can never do anything excellent; but by an excessive and undistinguishing thirst after it, you will come to have vulgar views; you will degrade your style; and your taste will be entirely corrupted. It is certain that the lowest style will be the most popular, as it falls within the compass of ignorance itself; and the vulgar will always be pleased with what is natural, in the confined and misunderstood sense of the word."

DISCOURSE VII.

"Whoever would reform a nation, supposing a bad taste to prevail in it, will not accomplish his purpose by going directly against the stream of their prejudices. Men's minds must be prepared to receive what is new to them. Reformation is a work of time. A national taste, however wrong it may be, cannot be totally changed at once; we must yield a little to the prepossession which has taken hold on the mind, and we may then bring people to adopt what would offend them, if endeavored to be introduced by violence."

DISCOURSE XII.

"Treatises on education and methods of study have always appeared to me to have one general fault. They proceed upon a false supposition of life; as if we possessed not only a power over events and circumstances, but had a greater power over ourselves than I believe any of us will be found to possess. Instead of supposing ourselves to be perfect patterns of wisdom and virtue, it seems to me more reasonable to treat ourselves (as I am sure we must now and then treat others) like humorsome children, whose fancies are often to be indulged in order to keep them in good humor with themselves and their pursuits."

DISCOURSE I.

" I must beg leave to submit one thing to the consideration of the visitors, which appears to me a matter of very great consequence, and the omission of which I think a principal defect in the method of education pursued in all the academies I have ever visited. The error I mean is, that the students never draw exactly from the living models which they have before them. It is not, indeed, their intention ; nor are they directed to do it. Their drawings resemble the model only in the attitude. They change the form according to their vague and uncertain ideas of beauty, and make a drawing rather of what they think the figure ought to be, than of what it appears. I have thought this the obstacle that has stopped the progress of many young men of real genius ; and I very much question whether a habit of drawing correctly what we see, will not give a proportionable power of drawing exactly what we imagine. He who endeavors to copy nicely the figure before him, not only acquires a habit of exactness and precision, but is continually advancing in his knowledge of the human figure ; and though he seems to superficial observers to make a slower progress, he will be found at last capable of adding (without running into capricious wildness) that grace and beauty, which is necessary to be given to his more finished works, and which cannot be got by the moderns, as it was not acquired by the ancients, but by an attentive and well-compared study of the human form."

DISCOURSE XII.

" However, I would not be understood to extend this doctrine to the younger students. The first part of the life of a student, like that of other school boys, must necessarily be a life of restraint. The grammar, the rudiments, however unpalatable, must at all events be mastered. After a habit is acquired of drawing correctly from the model (whatever it may be) which he has before him, the rest, I think, may be safely left to chance; always supposing that the student is *employed*, and that his studies are directed to the proper object."

Discourse XI.

" The properties of all objects, so far as a painter is concerned with them are, the outline or drawing, the color, and the light and shade. The drawing gives the forms ; the color, visible quality ; and the light and shade, its solidity.

" Excellence in any one of these parts of art will never be acquired by an artist, unless he has the habit of looking upon objects at large, and observing the effect which they have on the eye when it is dilated, and employed upon the whole, without seeing any of the parts distinctly. It is by this that we obtain the ruling characteristic, and that we learn to imitate it by short and dexterous methods. I do not mean by dexterity, a trick, or mechanical habit, formed by guess and established by custom; but that science which, by a profound knowledge of ends and means, discovers the shortest and surest way to its own purpose.

" If we examine with a critical view the manner of those painters whom we consider as patterns, we shall find that their great fame does not proceed from their works being more highly finished than those of other artists, or from a more minute attention to details, but from that enlarged comprehension which sees the whole object at once, and that energy of art which gives its characteristic effect by adequate expression."

Discourse XII.

" It is not uncommon to meet with artists who, from a long neglect of cultivating this intimacy with Nature, do not even know her when they see her; she appearing a stranger to them, from their being so habituated to their own representation of her. I have heard painters acknowledge, though in that acknowledgment no degradation of themselves was intended, that they could do better without Nature than with her; or, as they expressed it themselves, *that it only put them out.* A painter, with such ideas and such habits, is indeed in a most hopeless state. *The art of seeing Nature,* or, in other words, the art of using models, is in reality the great object, the point to which all our studies are directed. As for the power of being able to do tolerably well, from practice alone, let it be valued according to its worth. But I do not see in what manner it can be sufficient for the production of correct, excellent, and finished pictures. Works deserving this character never were produced, nor ever will arise, from memory alone; and I will venture to say, that an artist who brings to his work a mind tolerably furnished with the general principles of art, and a taste formed upon the works of good artists, in short, who knows in what excellence consists, will, with the assistance of models, which we will likewise suppose he has learned the art of using, be an over-match for the greatest painter that ever lived who should be debarred such advantages."

DISCOURSE X.

" What grace is, how it is acquired or conceived, are in speculation difficult questions: but *causa latet, res est notissima:* without any perplexing inquiry, the effect is hourly perceived. I shall only observe, that its natural foundation is correctness of design; and though grace may be sometimes united with incorrectness, it cannot proceed from it."

DISCOURSE XI.

" These observations may lead to very deep questions, which I do not mean here to discuss; among others, it may lead to an inquiry, why we are not always pleased with the most absolute possible resemblance of an imitation to its original object. Cases may exist in which such a resemblance may be even disagreeable. I shall only observe, that the effect of figures in wax-work, though certainly a more correct representation than can be given by painting or sculpture, is a sufficient proof that the pleasure we receive from imitation is not increased merely in proportion as it approaches to minute and detailed reality; we are pleased, on the contrary, by seeing ends accomplished by apparently inadequate means."

DISCOURSE III.

" I should be sorry, if what is here recommended should be at all understood to countenance a careless or undetermined manner of painting. For though the painter is to overlook the accidental discriminations of Nature, he is to exhibit distinctly, and with precision, the general forms of the great style in painting; and let me add, that he who possesses the knowledge of the exact form which every part of Nature ought to have, will be fond of expressing that knowledge with correctness and precision in all his works."

DEFINITIONS.

Aesthetics. The science which treats of the beautiful, and its various modes of representation in Nature and art ; the philosophy of the fine arts.

Accent. Emphasis of light or of dark in a light-and-shade drawing ; of dark in an outline drawing ; and of color or of light and dark in a color sketch.

Altitude. The perpendicular distance between the bases, or between the vertex and the base, of a solid or plane figure.

Angle. The difference in direction of two lines which meet or tend to meet. The lines are called the *sides*, and the point of meeting, the *vertex* of the angle.

An angle is measured by means of an arc of a circle described from its vertex as a centre and included between its sides. The centre of the arc is the vertex of the angle.

If the radius of the circle moves through $\frac{1}{360}$ of the circumference, it produces an angle which is taken as the unit for measuring angles, and is called a *degree*.

The degree is divided into sixty equal parts called *minutes*, and the minutes into sixty equal parts called *seconds*.

Degrees, minutes, and seconds are denoted by symbols. Thus 5 degrees, 13 minutes, 12 seconds, is written $5° \, 13' \, 12''$.

A RIGHT ANGLE is one which is formed by the radius moving through $\frac{1}{4}$ of the circumference. · It is an angle of 90°. A *straight* angle is formed when the radius has moved over $\frac{1}{2}$ of the circumference. It is an angle of 180°.

ACUTE ANGLE. An angle less than a right angle.

OBTUSE ANGLE. An angle greater than a right angle.

OBLIQUE ANGLE. One which is not a right or a straight angle.

REFLEX ANGLE.   One which is greater than 180°.

ADJACENT ANGLE.   Two angles are adjacent when they have the same vertex and a common side.

DIHEDRAL ANGLE.   The opening between two intersecting planes.

SOLID ANGLE.   One formed by planes which meet at a point.

Apex.   The summit or highest point of an object.

Appearance.   The image produced in the eye by the outline, light and shade, or color of any object.

Arc.   See Circle.

Arrangement.   The orderly disposition of objects or forms.

Axis of a Solid.   An imaginary straight line passing through its centre and about which the different parts are symmetrically arranged.

Axis of a Figure.   A straight line passing through the centre of a figure, and dividing it into two equal parts.

Axis of Symmetry.   A straight line so placed in a solid or a plane figure that every straight line meeting it at right angles and extending in each direction to the boundary of the solid or figure is bisected at the point of meeting.   In many solids and plane figures an axis of symmetry cannot be drawn.

Balance.   The equality of parts, obtained by the proper distribution of lines or of light and dark.

Base.   The opposite parallel polygons of prisms.   The polygon opposite the vertex of a pyramid.   The plane surfaces of cylinders and cones. The opposite parallel sides of a parallelogram or trapezoid.   The shortest or longest side of an isosceles triangle, and any side in any other triangle, but usually the lowest.

Bisect.   To divide into two equal parts.

Bisector.   A line which bisects.

Bisymmetrical.   Having one side the exact reverse of the other side.

Blend.   To soften and bring together.

Blocking-in Lines.   The lightest and simplest suggestions of the leading lines and masses of the subject.

Border.   Ornament, usually composed of units regularly repeated along a line.

Breadth. Simplicity due to large masses which subordinate details to the spirit and effect of the whole.

Chiaro-oscuro. The art of combining light and shade.

Cinquefoil. A figure composed of five leaf-like parts.

Circle. A plane figure bounded by a curved line, called a circumference, all points of which are equally distant from a point within called the *centre.*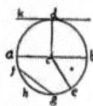

The boundary line is called the CIRCUMFERENCE.

DIAMETER. A straight line drawn through the centre, and connecting opposite points in the circumference, as *a b.*

RADIUS. The distance from its centre to the circumference, as *c e.*

SEMI-CIRCLE. Half a circle, formed by bisecting it with a diameter, as *a d b a.*

ARC. Any part of the circumference, as *e b.*

CHORD. A straight line whose ends are in the circumference, as *f g.*

SEGMENT. The part of a circle bounded by an arc and a chord, as *f h g f.*

SECTOR. The part of a circle bounded by two radii and an arc, as *b e c b.*

QUADRANT. A sector bounded by two radii and one fourth of the circumference, as *a c d a.*

TANGENT. A straight line which meets a circumference, but being produced does not cut it, as *k d.* The point of meeting is called the *point of contact* or *point of tangency.*

Circumscribe. A polygon is said to be circumscribed about a circle when each side of the polygon is a tangent to the circle ; and a circle is said to be circumscribed about a polygon when the circumference of the circle passes through all the vertices of the polygon.

Color. For color terms, see Color Manual.

Composition. The arrangement of the different lines, parts, and masses of a subject.

Concave. Curving inwardly.

Cone. A solid bounded by a plane surface called the *base*, which is a circle, ellipse, or other curved figure, and by a lateral surface which is everywhere curved, and tapers to a point called the *vertex*. Its base names the cone. Thus a circular cone is one whose base is a circle.

A RIGHT CIRCULAR CONE is generated by an isosceles triangle which revolves about its altitude as an axis. The equal sides of the triangle in any position are called *elements* of the surface. The length of an element is called the *slant height* of the cone. Unless otherwise stated "cone" means a right circular cone.

A FRUSTUM OF A CONE is the part included between the base and a plane parallel to the base and cutting all the elements of the cone.

A TRUNCATED CONE is the part included between the base and a plane oblique to the base and cutting all the elements of the cone.

Concentric. Having a common centre.

Conic Section. A section obtained by cutting a cone by a plane.

Construction. The making of any object.

Construction Lines. The lines by which the desired result is obtained.

Constructive Drawing. A drawing intended for the workman who is to make the object.

Contour. The outline of the general appearance of an object.

Contour Element. An element which is in the contour of an object.

Contrast. The effect due to the juxtaposition of different lines, different forms, different masses of light and dark, or different colors.

Conventionalization. In art, the expression of the spirit and important truths of Nature by a subordination of less important features.

Convergence. Lines extending toward a common point, or planes extending toward a common line.

Convex. Rising or swelling into a spherical or rounded form.

Corner. The point of meeting of the edges of a solid, or of two sides of a plane figure.

Crescent. A figure of the shape of the new moon.

Cross. Two bars, or parts, intersecting or crossing each other in various ways. The symbol of the Christian religion.

Greek Cross.   Latin Cross.   Maltese Cross.   St. Andrew's Cross.

Cross-hatched. In mechanical drawing, a half tinting placed upon parts cut by a cutting plane. In free-hand drawing, the use of lines crossing each other and producing light and shade effects.

Curvature. Variation from straightness.

Curve. A line of which no part is straight.

> REVERSED. One whose curvature is first in one direction and then in the opposite direction.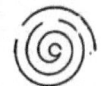

> SPIRAL. A plane curve which winds about and recedes, according to some law, from its point of beginning, which is called its *centre*.

Cylinder. A solid bounded by a curved surface and·by two opposite faces called bases ; the bases may be ellipses, circles, or other curved figures, and name the cylinder. Thus a circular cylinder (the ordinary form) is one whose bases are circles.

> A RIGHT CIRCULAR CYLINDER is generated by the revolution of a rectangle about one side as an axis. The side about which the rectangle revolves is called the *height* of the cylinder, also its *axis*. The side opposite the axis describes the curved surface of the cylinder, and in any of its positions is called an *element* of the surface.

Cylindrical. Having the general form of a cylinder.

Degree. The 360th part of a circumference of a circle.

Describe. To make or draw a curved line.

Design. Any arrangement or combination to produce desired results in industry or art.

Develop. To unroll or lay out upon one plane the surface of an object

Diagonal. A straight line in any polygon which connects vertices not adjacent.

In regular polygons, diagonals are called *long* when they pass through the centre, as *c d*, and *short* when they extend between parallel sides, as *a b*.

Diameter. See Circle. In a regular polygon with an even number of sides a line joining the centres of two opposite sides is often called a diameter.

Diverging Lines. Lines extending from a common point.

Edge. The intersection of any two surfaces. The boundary line. Edges are straight or curved, and are represented by lines.

Elevation. A drawing made on a vertical plane by means of projecting lines perpendicular to the plane from the points of the object. The terms elevation, vertical projection, and front view all have the same meaning.

Ellipse. A plane figure bounded by a line such that the sum of the distances of any point in it, as *c*, from two given points *e* and *f*, called *foci*, is equal to a given line, as *a b*. The point midway between the foci is called the *centre*.

> The TRANSVERSE AXIS of an ellipse is the longest diameter that can be drawn in it, as *a b*. It is also called the *major* or *long* axis.
>
> The CONJUGATE AXIS is the shortest diameter which can be drawn, as *c d*. It is also called the *minor* or *short* axis. The foci, *e* and *f*, are two points in the long diameter whose distance from *c* or *d* is equal to one-half *a b*.

Face. One of the plane surfaces of a solid. It may be bounded by straight or curved edges.

Finishing. Completing a drawing, whose lines have been determined, by erasing unnecessary lines and strengthening and accenting where this is required.

Foreshortening. Apparent decrease in length, due to a position oblique (or parallel) to the visual rays.

Free Arm Movement. Movement of the arm from the shoulder.

Free-hand. Executed by the hand, without the aid of instruments.

Fret. A band or border composed of lines forming a succession of angles and often interlacing.

Frustum. See Cone and Pyramid.

Generated. Produced by.

Geometric. According to geometry.

Gradation. A gradual change from light to dark, or from one color to another.

Half-tint. The shading produced by means of parallel equidistant lines.

Hemisphere. Half a sphere, obtained by bisecting a sphere by a plane.

Horizon. In pictorial art, a horizontal line at the level of the eye.

Horizontal. Parallel to the surface of smooth water.

In drawings, a line parallel to the top and bottom of the sheet is called horizontal.

Inscribe. A polygon is said to be inscribed in a circle when all its vertices are in the circumference of the circle ; and a circle is said to be inscribed in a polygon when the circumference of the circle is touched by each side of the polygon.

Instrumental. By the use of instruments.

Interlacing. The arrangement of one part of a design so that it passes alternately above and below another part.

Lateral Surface. The surface of a solid excluding the base or bases.

Level of the Eye. The level or position of a horizontal plane passing through the spectator's eye.

Line. A line has length only. In a drawing its representation has width but is called a line.

STRAIGHT. One which has the same direction throughout its entire length.

CURVED. One no part of which is straight.

BROKEN. One composed of different successive straight lines.

MIXED. One composed of straight and curved lines.

CENTRE. A line used to indicate the centre of an object.

CONSTRUCTION. A working line used to obtain required lines.

DOTTED. A line composed of short dashes.

DASH. A line composed of long dashes.

DOT and DASH. A line composed of dots and dashes alternating.

DIMENSION. A line upon which a dimension is placed.

FULL. An unbroken line, usually representing a visible edge.

SHADOW. A line about twice as wide as the ordinary full line.

A straight line is often called simply a line, and a curved line, a curve.

Longitudinal. In the direction of the length of an object.

Model. *A form used for study.

Oblique. Neither horizontal nor vertical.

Oblong. A rectangle with unequal sides.

Ornament. Decorative arrangement of line, light and shade, color, or relief.

HISTORIC. That designed in previous ages.

Oval. A plane figure resembling the longitudinal section of an egg ; or elliptical in shape.

Overall. The entire length.

Ovoid. An egg-shaped solid.

Parallel. Having the same direction and everywhere equally distant.

Parallelogram. See Quadrilateral.

Pattern. That which is used as a guide or copy in making anything.

FLAT. One made of paper or other thin material.

SOLID. One which reproduces the form and size of the object to be made.

Perimeter. The boundary of a closed plane figure.

Perpendicular. At an angle of 90°.

Perspective. The art of making upon a plane, called the *picture plane,* such a representation of objects that the lines of the drawing appear to coincide with those of the object, when the eye is at one fixed point called the *station point.*

DIAGRAM. An exact perspective drawing obtained scientifically by perspective methods. It is often very false pictorially when not seen from the station point.

PARALLEL. Diagram perspective which represents a cubical form by the use of one vanishing point, and represents by its real shape any face parallel to the picture plane.

ANGULAR. Diagram perspective in which two sets of horizontal edges of a cubical form are at angles to the picture plane, and the object is thus represented by the use of two vanishing points.

OBLIQUE. Diagram perspective in which, none of the edges of a cubical form being parallel to the picture plane, it is represented by the use of three vanishing points.

FREE-HAND or MODEL DRAWING. A drawing which, without confining the eye to the station point, represents as far as possible the actual appearance of objects. It is made free-hand, and is for most purposes more satisfactory than an exact diagram perspective.

Plan. Plan, horizontal projection, and top view have the same meaning, and designate the representation of an object made on a horizontal plane by means of vertical projecting lines. In architecture it means a horizontal section.

Plane Figure. A part of a plane surface bounded by lines.

A plane figure is called *rectilinear* if bounded by straight lines, *curvilinear* if bounded by curved lines, and *mixtilinear* if bounded by both straight and curved lines.

Similar figures are those that have the same shape.

Plinth. A cylinder or prism, whose axis is its least dimension. It is *circular, triangular, square,* etc., according as it has circles, triangles, squares, etc., for bases.

Polygon. A plane figure bounded by straight lines.

An EQUILATERAL POLYGON is one whose sides are all equal.

An EQUIANGULAR POLYGON is one whose angles are all equal.

A REGULAR POLYGON is one which is equilateral and equiangular.

PARALLEL POLYGONS are those whose sides are respectively parallel.

TRIANGLE.   A polygon having three sides (1).

QUADRILATERAL.   A polygon having four sides (2).

PENTAGON.   A polygon having five sides (3).

HEXAGON.   A polygon having six sides (4).

HEPTAGON.   A polygon having seven sides (5).

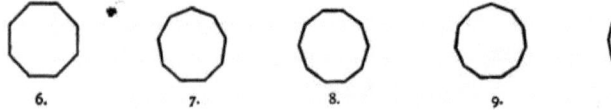

6.   7.   8.   9.   10.

OCTAGON.   A polygon having eight sides (6).

NONAGON.   A polygon having nine sides (7).

DECAGON.   A polygon having ten sides (8).

UNDECAGON.   A polygon having eleven sides (9).

DODECAGON.   A polygon having twelve sides (10).

The centre of a regular polygon is the common intersection of perpendiculars erected at the middle points of its sides.

The polygons represented in the figures are regular polygons.

A **Polyhedron** is a solid bounded by planes.   It is regular when its faces are regular equal polygons.

There can be but five regular polyhedrons :

1. The TETRAHEDRON, or PYRAMID, which has four triangular faces.

2. The HEXAHEDRON, or CUBE, which has six square faces.

3. The OCTAHEDRON, which has eight triangular faces.

4. The DODECAHEDRON, which has twelve pentagonal faces.

5. The ICOSAHEDRON, which has twenty triangular faces.

The term hexahedron is applied only to a regular polyhedron : the other terms may be applied to irregular polyhedrons.

An infinite number of irregular polyhedrons, also an infinite number of other solids bounded by plane or curved surfaces, may be conceived.

Prism. A solid bounded by two equal parallel polygons, having their equal sides parallel, and by three or more parallelograms.

The polygons are called the *bases* of the prism, the parallelograms the *lateral faces*, the intersections of the lateral faces, the *lateral edges*.

Prisms are called *triangular, square, pentagonal*, etc., according as the bases are triangles, squares, pentagons, etc.

A RIGHT PRISM is one in which the edges connecting the bases are perpendicular to the bases.

An OBLIQUE PRISM is one in which the edges connecting the bases are not perpendicular to the bases.

A REGULAR PRISM is a right prism whose bases are regular polygons.

A TRUNCATED PRISM is the part of a prism included between the base and a section made by a plane inclined to the base, and cutting all the lateral edges.

The ALTITUDE of a prism is the perpendicular distance between the bases.

The AXIS of a regular prism is a straight line connecting the centres of its bases.

A RIGHT SECTION of a prism is a section made by a plane perpendicular to its lateral edges.

A PARALLELOPIPED is a prism whose bases are parallelograms.

Produce. To continue or extend.

Profile. The contour outline of an object.

Projection. Orthographic. The view or representation of an object obtained upon a plane by projecting lines perpendicular to the plane.

Pyramid. A solid of which one face, called the *base*, is a polygon, and the other faces, called *lateral faces*, are triangles having a common vertex called the *vertex* of the pyramid. The intersections of the lateral faces are called the *lateral edges*.

A pyramid is called *triangular, square*, etc., according as its base is a triangle, square, etc.

A REGULAR PYRAMID is one whose base is a regular polygon and whose vertex is in a perpendicular erected at the centre of the base. Its other faces are equal isosceles triangles. The altitude of any of these triangles is called the *slant height* of the pyramid.

A FRUSTUM of a pyramid is the part included between the base and a plane parallel to the base and cutting all the *lateral* edges.

A TRUNCATED PYRAMID is the part included between the base and a plane oblique to the base and cutting all the *lateral* edges.

The AXIS of a pyramid is a straight line connecting the vertex and the centre of the base.

The ALTITUDE of a pyramid is the perpendicular distance from the vertex to the base.

Quadrant. See Circle.

Quadrilateral. A plane figure bounded by four straight lines. These lines are the *sides*. The angles formed by the lines are the *angles*, and the vertices of these angles are the *vertices* of the quadrilateral.

A PARALLELOGRAM is a quadrilateral which has its opposite sides parallel.

A TRAPEZIUM is a quadrilateral which has no two sides parallel.

A TRAPEZOID is a quadrilateral which has two sides, and only two sides, parallel.

A RECTANGLE is a quadrilateral whose angles are right angles.

A SQUARE is a rectangle whose sides are equal.

A RHOMBOID is a parallelogram whose angles are oblique angles.

A RHOMBUS is a rhomboid whose sides are equal.

The side upon which a parallelogram stands and the opposite side are called respectively its lower and upper bases.

Quadrisect. To divide into four equal parts.

Quatrefoil. A figure composed of four leaf-like parts.

Radiation. Proceeding from a common point or line.

Reflected Light. The light seen on the shadow side of any object, and reflected from some other object.

Relation. The harmony or contrast of form, value, or color.

Rendering or Handling. The way in which a medium is used.

Repetition. The arrangement of a unit on a line, around a centre, about a line as axis, or upon geometric lines covering a surface.

Representation. Any kind of drawing, painting, or sculpture.

Retreating. Going away from.

Rosette. Arrangement of petal-like units about a centre.

Section. A projection upon a plane parallel to a cutting plane which intersects any object. The section generally represents the part behind the cutting plane, and represents the cut surfaces by cross-hatching.

Sectional. Showing the section made by a plane.

Sector and Segment. See Circle.

Shadow. Shade and shadow have about the same meaning, as generally used ; but it will be well to designate by shadow those parts of an object which are turned away from the direct rays of light, while those surfaces which receive less direct rays and are intermediate in value between the light and the shadow are called shade surfaces.

> CAST. The shadow projected on any body or surface by some other body.

Similar Figures are those which have the same shape.

Solid. A solid has three dimensions, length, breadth, and thickness. It may be bounded by plane surfaces, by curved surfaces, or by both plane and curved surfaces. As commonly understood, a solid is a limited portion of space filled with matter, but geometry does not consider the matter and deals simply with the shapes and sizes of solids.

Sphere. A solid bounded by a curved surface every point of which is equally distant from a point within called the centre.

A sphere may be generated by the revolution of a circle about a diameter as an axis.

Spheroid (Ellipsoid). A solid generated by the revolution of an ellipse about either diameter. When revolved about the long diameter, the spheroid is called *prolate* or the long spheroid; when about the short diameter, it is called *oblate* or the flat spheroid. The earth is an oblate spheroid.

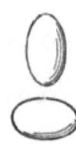

Spiral. See Curve.

Stippling. Filling in the space between hatching lines, or producing an effect, by means of dots.

Surface. The boundary of a solid. It has but two dimensions, length and breadth.

Surfaces are plane or curved.

> A PLANE SURFACE is one upon which a straight line can be drawn in any direction.

> A CURVED SURFACE is one no part of which is plane.

The surface of the sphere is curved in every direction, while the curved surfaces of the cylinder and cone are straight in one direction.

The surface of a solid is no part of the solid, but is simply the boundary of the solid. It has two dimensions only, and any number of surfaces put together will give no thickness.

Symbolism. The use of conventional forms to suggest ideas not inherent in the forms.

Symmetry. *Design.* A proper adjustment or adaptation of parts to one another and to the whole.

> BILATERAL. Having two parts in exact reverse of each other.

Symmetry. *Geometry.* If a solid can be divided by a plane into two parts such that every straight line, perpendicular to the plane and extending from the plane in each direction to the surface of the solid, is bisected by the plane, the solid is called a *symmetrical* solid, and the plane is called a *plane of symmetry*. If two planes of symmetry can be drawn in a solid, their intersection is called an *axis of symmetry*. See Axis of Symmetry.

The line about which a plane figure revolves when it generates a solid of revolution is an axis of symmetry for the solid; it is also called the *axis of revolution*.

Tangent. A straight line and a curved line, or two curved lines, are tangent when they have one point common and cannot intersect; lines or surfaces are tangent to curved surfaces when they have one point or one line common and cannot intersect.

Technique. The handling or way in which an effect is obtained.

Texture. The character of a surface.

Trefoil. A figure composed of three leaf-like parts.

Triangle. A plane figure bounded by three straight lines. These lines are called the *sides.* The angles that they form are called the *angles* of the triangle, and the vertices of these angles, the *vertices* of the triangle.

Triangles are named by their sides and angles.

A SCALENE TRIANGLE is one in which no two sides are equal.

An ISOSCELES TRIANGLE is one in which two sides are equal.

An EQUILATERAL TRIANGLE is one in which the three sides are equal.

A RIGHT TRIANGLE is one in which one of the angles is a right angle.

An OBTUSE TRIANGLE is one in which one of the angles is obtuse.

An ACUTE TRIANGLE is one in which all the angles are acute.

The HYPOTENUSE is the side of a right triangle opposite the right angle. The other sides are called the *legs.*

An EQUIANGULAR TRIANGLE is one in which the three angles are equal. The value of each angle is 60°.

The BASE is the side on which the triangle is supposed to stand. In an isosceles triangle, the equal sides are called the *legs*, the other side the *base;* in other triangles any one of the sides may be called the base.

The ALTITUDE is the perpendicular distance from the vertex to the base. Except in the isosceles triangle, there are three altitudes.

The vertex of the angle opposite the base is often called the *vertex* of the triangle.

Trisect. To divide into three equal parts.

Truncated. A truncated solid is the part of a solid included between the base and a plane cutting the solid oblique to the base.

Type Form. A perfect geometrical plane figure or solid.

Unit of Design. The figure repeated in a design or arrangement.

Value. In color the relative amount of light contained in different colors. The strongest value is the lightest.

As used by artists the word generally means the difference in effect due to any cause whatever, as light, color, shadow, atmosphere, etc.

A flat value is one with no gradation.

Variety. The effect due to the combination of parts which are not alike.

Vertical. Upright or perpendicular to a horizontal plane or line.

Vertical and perpendicular are not synonymous terms.

Vertex. See Angle, Quadrilateral, Triangle. The vertex of a solid is the point in which its axis intersects the lateral surface.

View. See Elevation. Views are called front, top, right or left side, back, or bottom, according as they are made on the different planes of projection. They are also sometimes named according to the part of the object shown, as edge view, end view, or face view.

Working Drawing. One which gives all the information necessary to enable the workman to construct the object.

Working Lines. See Lines.